What people are saying about
Is Lap Band Surgery for Me?

It's rare to find a book that is written for patients by patients. In *Is Lap Band Surgery for Me? Your Step-by-Step Guide to Lasting Weight Loss*, Gloria and Sandi combine their knowledge and experience to make your decision less intimidating.

—Jessica T, RN, BSN, CBN

I wish all of the weight loss surgery patients that I've seen could have started by following this step-by-step guide…

—Frank G, Program Coordinator
St. John's Center for Surgical Weight Loss

Thank you again for that wonderful information. It has helped in getting me ready to be banded.

—Pamela W

Thank you for sharing your stories and experiences and encouraging us who are still early in the process! I couldn't believe how difficult it was to find something not written by the band companies…

—Chris W

The two wonderful women who wrote this book are great resources. If you can see yourself accepting and making the changes they explain, it is worth everything!!

—Meg G

This is great. The more help we can get for the world out there the better.
—Nancy K-B, Bariatric Patient Support Facilitator

Soon, my dears…I will be living the dream like you are!!! You ROCK!!! Thank you!
—Angie V

Thanks so much for sharing such exciting and encouraging words with us. I know exactly where I want to be a year from now.

—Rosemary S

Is Lap Band Surgery for Me?

Your Step-by-Step Guide to Lasting Weight Loss

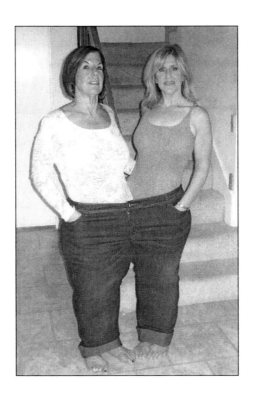

Sandi Henderson and Gloria Samuels

Published by Wheatmark®
610 East Delano Street, Suite 104, Tucson, Arizona 85705 U.S.A.
www.wheatmark.com

ISBN: 978-1-60494-494-5
LCCN: 2010934800

This book is dedicated to the millions of people throughout the world who have been battling with obesity throughout their lives. If we succeed in generating hope in one person, then this work has been more than worth our time and energy. We have come to know, through our own personal experiences, that obesity is not a moral failure but is rather a problem requiring medical intervention. This medical intervention has allowed both of us to finally achieve and maintain what had eluded us for most of our lives: a normal, healthy weight. We want to share with you what we have learned on our journeys.

—Sandi and Gloria

Foreword

Bariatric surgery is an immensely rewarding field of medicine. I have had the opportunity to help patients transform their lives for the better and to reach goals that had seemed beyond achievable. As a surgeon who has performed thousands of weight loss operations, I have seen lap band surgery become increasingly popular since first being approved in the United States in 2001. But why is it that some patients succeed while others struggle? In my practice, I've learned a lot about what makes a successful weight loss surgery patient. Patients who do their homework, establish a plan, and embark upon this journey with their eyes wide open improve their chances of success. That is what this book is all about.

What you will find here is very different than what you typically get from your surgeon. This is not a medical book; this is a journey of self-exploration. It is filled with valuable exercises, information, and real-life experiences. It's a step-by-step journey guided by two people who have achieved and maintained outstanding results with their lap bands, two people who understand that the band is a tool and know how to use it. Sandi and Gloria are your peers. They know what it takes to be successful, and they can help you develop your plan.

By using this book, you can develop a clear and thorough understanding of how to use your lap band as a tool and find out what's in store for you should you decide to proceed with surgery. It's time to get serious; weight loss surgery is not a magic bullet. This book captures candid experiences, gives you an honest picture of the facts, and shows you how to optimize your lap band results. Sandi and Gloria simplify the process of understanding how to achieve your goals so you can understand what to expect and what it will take to be successful forever.

The lap band operation by itself is not enough to allow you to achieve your goals. To think that you will achieve your goals just by having an operation is delusional. It takes more than a few adjustments and a feeling of being full to achieve lasting weight loss results. Your ability to use your lap band to its full potential is increased when you surround yourself with other successful people. You need the facts. You need to know that your surgeon will perform the operation and work with you to adjust your band—but you need to do the work. The band can help you with portion control, hunger, and satiety. The rest is up to you. Not everyone is prepared to do what it takes. There are some patients who are too set in their ways to achieve the results they are looking for and some who are not willing to put in the effort it will take to get there. To achieve optimal results, the responsibility is yours. You must become empowered to achieve your goals. The band will not do it for you. The doctor will not do it for you. You must do it for you. And this book can help you understand what that means.

The book *Outliers* by Malcolm Gladwell is a study of what it takes to be successful. To be a true expert in anything requires thousands of hours of work. It takes practice. There is no substitute for hard work and effort. There is no easy way out when someone wants to become an expert at managing his or her weight. It takes practice and desire to reach success.

Weight loss surgery is no different. So you must ask yourself some questions before entering into this process: How much do you want to lose weight? What are your goals? Are your goals realistic? How much work are you willing to put in to achieve those goals? What is your strategy? What is your plan? How are you going to practice weight loss? How are you going to use this tool?

Patients learn best from their peers. Gloria and Sandi have done extensive research and talked to hundreds of patients to bring together a comprehensive resource that is honest, uplifting, and invaluable to anyone considering weight loss surgery. Gloria and Sandi are real patients. They are among the most successful long-term lap band patients. This book fills a gap in information. It is an easy-to-understand, step-by-step process to guide you through your decision to answer the question: Is lap band surgery for me?

The lap band system and surgery works. Learning how to use this tool properly is the challenge. Patients can be successful once they learn how this tool helps them achieve their goals.

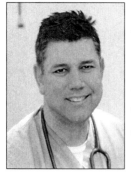

Helmuth T. Billy, MD
Ventura Advanced Surgical Associates
Ventura, California
www.drbillybariatrics.com

Dr. Billy is the leading lap band and laparoscopic gastric bypass surgeon in Ventura and Santa Barbara County and has performed thousands of bariatric surgeries. Dr. Billy is currently the director of Bariatric Surgery at St. John's Regional Medical Center located in Oxnard, California, a recognized bariatric Center of Excellence.

Dr. Billy obtained his undergraduate degree in Molecular Biology at the University of California, Berkeley. He subsequently received his medical degree at the University of California, Davis, School of Medicine. Dr. Billy received additional training in the techniques of the lap band system prior to its release by the FDA in 2001. He is actively involved as a teaching faculty member for placement of the LAP-BAND® System and has educated and proctored dozens of surgeons throughout the West as part of their educational training. Dr. Billy has been a faculty member at numerous national educational events and surgeon training workshops. He has been a featured speaker at the annual meeting of the American Society of Metabolic and Bariatric Surgery and was a contributing author on the recently released SAGES Bariatric Surgery Manual published by the Society of Alimentary and Gastroendoscopic Surgeons. Dr. Billy has an international reputation and has lectured and taught principles of bariatric surgery in Mexico, Taiwan, and India.

Acknowledgments

This book has its roots back in January 2004 when Sandi Henderson first attended a weight loss surgery seminar. It continued to develop through August 2006 when Gloria Samuels had her lap band surgery, and then was finally given life in September 2009 when Banded Living™ LLC was born. None of this could have happened without the encouragement, surgical skill, support, and guidance of Dr. Helmuth T. Billy and his incredible staff. Dr. Billy and his staff supported us throughout our weight loss journeys and have been incredibly encouraging of our desire to pay it forward with this book, our membership website, and all of our individual endeavors. Dr. Billy has been our advisor throughout the development of this book, freely giving his time, insights, and experience to make suggestions, as well as to cheer us along. Jessica Thorpe, RN, BSN, CBN invested her limited personal time to edit this book and make invaluable suggestions regarding content and approach. Sara Reyes, RN, BSN, CBN gave her valuable time reviewing our basic concept (by patients, for patients) and making suggestions. For their time, energy, and honest advice, we thank them all.

Throughout our weight loss journeys, the conception of Banded Living, and the writing, editing, and publishing of this book—with all its angst and ups and downs—we had two men constantly by our sides: our husbands. For their unwavering support, candid insights, and belief in us, we are eternally grateful.

Our children and grandchildren have been consistently patient with our unavailability because we had to work on this book. We can only hope that the lessons of dedication and perseverance in reaching for and achieving goals were lessons that did not come at too high an expense to our families. We also hope that through this journey they have learned to do as we do—live a healthy lifestyle.

Let's not forget the hundreds of other patients we've met along this journey, whose tips, personal stories, laughter, and tears have helped inspire and propel us. We also want to recognize the many friends who cheered us along.

Finally, without the courage that each of us individually demonstrated to choose lap band surgery and choose "results not typical" as our goals, we could not have written this book that we offer to you, our readers, as a guide to deciding what the right path is for you on your journey to health, well being, and lasting weight loss.

Medical Disclaimer

The information provided in this book (including all text, graphics, and images) is for informational purposes only. It is not intended to be construed, nor should the reader construe it as, medical care or medical advice, and it is not a replacement for medical care given by physicians or trained medical personnel. Readers should always seek the advice of their physicians or other qualified healthcare providers when experiencing symptoms or health problems, or when investigating the possibility of treatment. The authors are patients, not physicians, and speak only of their personal experiences and about the information they have gathered over time.

It is the reader's responsibility to evaluate the information and results from information provided by the authors. Readers should not use the information contained in this book to diagnose or treat a medical or health condition. Readers should consult their physicians in all matters relating to their health, and particularly in respect to any symptoms that may require diagnosis or medical attention.

Banded Living, LLC and its members, managers, officers, employees, consultants, and representatives specifically disclaim all responsibility for any liability, loss, or risk, personal or otherwise, that is incurred as a consequence, directly or indirectly, of the use or application of any of the material in this book. Banded Living, LLC, is not responsible for any inaccuracies, omissions, or editorial errors, or for any consequences resulting from the information provided. By continuing to read this book, the reader indicates an understanding and acceptance of the terms in this medical disclaimer.

Contents

Introduction

Why This Book?

If you have picked up this book, undoubtedly we have three things in common:

1. You have a serious weight issue.
2. Your way of trying to lose weight hasn't worked.
3. You want to learn more about lap band surgery.

When we, the authors of this book, first started exploring lap band surgery, it was very difficult to find honest, unbiased information. Patients with long-term success were hard to come by. Figuring out whether or not to have weight loss surgery and deciding which surgery to have was very confusing and highly intimidating.

Today, that process is still very confusing. This book fills that gap. There is a lot of conflicting information on the Internet from many well-intentioned (and sometimes not so well-intentioned) sources, as well as from advertising by the weight loss industry. Friends and family may also have opinions based on old information, which can further add to your confusion. This is why we wrote this book.

We are very disheartened when we hear about people who have "failed" with lap band surgery. Failure can mean many things: not achieving the average weight loss, not achieving your goals, not achieving someone else's goals for you. In our experience, the most successful patients are those who go into surgery with their eyes wide open, with realistic expectations and a plan. All too often we hear, "I had a surgery; it was supposed to work. But I didn't know I would have to…"

This book is an easy-to-follow, step-by-step guide that will help you answer the question:

"Is lap band surgery for me?" We will take you through a journey of self-discovery so that you can answer that question for yourself. If you choose to proceed, you will know how the lap band works and what it takes to achieve success with lap band surgery; you will know what to expect and what you need to do. And if you choose not to have lap band surgery, you will know why.

This book is *not* designed to sell you on lap band surgery. It is designed to help you understand what you need to know to be a successful lap band patient.

For those who decide to move forward with surgery, you will be going in with your eyes wide open. Your completed book will be a useful tool that you can refer to again and again throughout your journey. It will become part of your lap band toolkit.

How This Book Is Organized—The Step-by-Step Process

This book is organized into seven simple, easy-to-follow steps. Each step is a chapter with goals, information, real-life patient perspectives, and exercises. You can see a visual representation of these steps below:

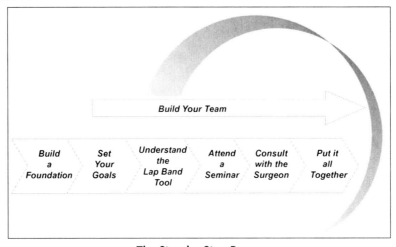

The Step-by-Step Process

Step 1: Build a Foundation

In this step you research the facts. Lap band surgery is not for everyone, and you need the facts—including the benefits, risks, complications, and long-term results—in order to make an informed decision. You will become familiar with who should consider weight loss surgery and learn about common weight loss surgery options. You will be able to determine if you fit within the National Institute of Health (NIH) guidelines and if you may be considered a candidate for weight loss surgery. You will also be provided with resources to get the most up-to-date information.

Step 2: Build Your Team

This step is ongoing; you will add to your team throughout your journey. The goal of this step is to build the best team possible so that you can surround yourself with people who will help you be successful. You need to understand what support you will or won't get from the people closest to you. Your team includes your family and loved ones, your primary care physician, the bariatric surgical practice you choose, other patients, and your friends and colleagues.

Step 3: Set Your Goals

This step will help you to establish realistic goals for lap band surgery in terms of health, weight, and quality of life.

Step 4: Understand the Lap Band Tool

The goal of this step is to be able to understand why lap band surgery is different than all the diets you've been on. You will learn how the band works, what "restriction" means, and how successful patients use this tool. You will understand the role of aftercare and understand your eating habits and what you need to change. Most importantly, this step will help you understand what you need to do to be a successful lap band patient.

Step 5: Attend a Seminar

Most surgical practices offer free informational seminars. This step will help you get the most from that seminar. Once you have the facts and have begun to understand the lap band tool, you will have positioned yourself to get the most from these free informational seminars. The seminar is a great way to learn more about lap band surgery and about your prospective surgeon and his or her program. It may also be an opportunity to meet other patients and staff from the surgeon's practice.

Step 6: Consult with the Surgeon

If you make it this far, you are probably seriously considering getting a lap band. This step will help you prepare for your consultation. It will also help you assess what you learned during the consultation. This is your opportunity to get your specific questions answered and learn more about the surgeon and his or her practice. People who have lap bands need to see their doctor often, especially during the first year. You need to determine if the practice is for you.

Step 7: Put It All Together

This final step will guide you through putting it all together so that you can answer the question: "Is lap band surgery for me?" You will be in a position to make an informed decision grounded in facts and realistic expectations. If you chose to proceed with surgery, you will be well informed and prepared to be a successful lap band patient. If you decide not to proceed, you will know why.

About the Exercises in This Book

These exercises are designed for *you*. You will only get out of them what you put into them. Being honest is the only way to truly uncover what you need to know. This is *your* book. You owe it to yourself to invest fully in the process.

How to Use This Book

This book follows a sequential process. It's a very sensible process. However, not everyone starts at the beginning. For example, your first step may have been to attend a free informational seminar, yet you may still be struggling to understand how the lap band tool works from a patient's perspective. In that case you may want to start with step 4: Understand the Lap Band Tool.

Depending upon where you are in your own journey, you may decide not to start at the beginning of this book. That's fine; you need to find what works best for you. We do, however, strongly encourage you to go through all of the exercises to make sure you haven't missed anything that may be important to your decision or your success.

This book is designed so that you can take it with you to meetings and doctor appointments. By the time you make your decision, it should be well worn with lots of notes. For those who have planned a wedding or had a baby, you can use it like a wedding planner or baby book to document your journey, keep notes, and jot down questions. It's your book, and this is your story.

Good luck on your journey! Here's to your success, whatever you decide is right for you.

About Banded Living

Banded Living is about *living* life to the fullest, free from the burdens of obesity. Banded Living is a community by lap band patients for lap band patients, including people exploring lap band surgery and those who have had surgery and want to use their tool to get the best results.

The Banded Living community is your lap band community regardless of who made your band, how much it holds, or where you had your surgery. We all have had similar experiences and challenges, but our journeys are different from those who have had other types of weight loss surgery.

Since our surgeries, we (Sandi and Gloria) have maintained a combined weight loss of 340 pounds. Together we have over ten years of experience as patients and as mentors to others with lap bands. We are passionate about giving back and helping others conquer obesity. We are not doctors and don't give medical advice; we encourage you to work closely with your doctor, just as we have with ours. As new information becomes available, please be sure to look for updates on bandedliving.com.

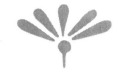

Sandi's Story

I have been fighting the fat war since I was four years old. I finally won the war, leaving only small skirmishes that crop up occasionally. My friends tell me these little battles are what a "normal" person always deals with.

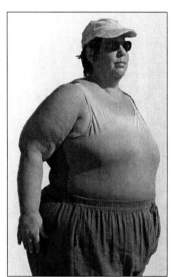

Sandi before lap band surgery

Just six years ago, I weighed 424 pounds, had arthritis in my right knee, and had trouble walking across a parking lot. My asthma would force me to stop and catch my breath several times. I rented a scooter to be able to take my grandkids to Disneyland. I let my husband go into the market while I waited in the truck. People looked fearfully at me when I got on a plane, hoping I wasn't sitting next to them. In March 2004, I had a hypertension crisis that got my attention. To that point, my arthritis, asthma, reflux, and sleep apnea had not yet been enough to make me take notice.

I have succeeded at most everything I have tried in life—I have a wonderful marriage of more than forty years to my soul mate, a great daughter, awesome grandchildren, and a successful business that I built from scratch over twenty years ago. But I could never get a handle on my weight for longer than five minutes.

On May 28, 2004, at fifty-five years old, I had life-changing—and life-saving—lap band surgery. Within twenty-eight months I had lost 250 pounds. Now, more than six years after the surgery, I am holding at 175 pounds and loving it. I am off all my medications and move freely and

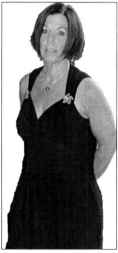

Sandi after lap band surgery

vigorously throughout my new life.

　　With the help of this tool and a great support team, I have reached a place in life where it is fun to go anywhere and try new things, and I actually enjoy looking at pictures of myself (well, most of the time). You will read more about me and my personal journey throughout this book.

Step 1: Build a Foundation

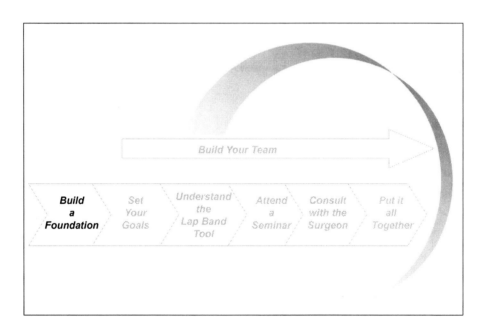

Objectives

The objectives of this step are to guide you to be able to:

- Understand the growing problem of obesity
- Understand who should consider weight loss surgery
- Become familiar with common weight loss surgeries
- Determine if you would be considered a candidate for lap band surgery

Introduction: Searching for that Magic Wand

With the growing obesity epidemic in the United States, there is a lot of research underway aimed at the obesity problem. Many of us are still hoping for a magic wand—something that will finally make this weight loss battle disappear forever. It is generally accepted that obesity in humans is a complex problem, which creates a challenge for researchers. I'm still hoping for a magic wand, but for now I'm thrilled to have my band.

—Gloria

The information in this book is current as of the time of printing and provides a foundation of information for anyone exploring lap band surgery. The source material for this section includes:

- The National Institute of Health, Weight Information Network, Publication number 08-4006, March 2009
- Cleveland Clinic Journal of Medicine, Volume 73, Number In Press 2006
  Journal American Medical Association June 2009
- http://www.lapband.com
- http://www.realize.com

At the end of this section you will also find a list of websites for some of the most current information.

The Growing Problem of Obesity

Over two-thirds of adults in the United States are overweight, and over one-third are obese, according to data from the National Health and Nutrition Examination Survey 2007–2008. In addition, approximately 15 million Americans are classified as morbidly obese. The cost to the U.S. health care system for obesity is estimated at over $150 billion annually.

But what do *overweight* and *obese* really mean? Overweight specifically refers to an excessive amount of body weight that may come from muscles, bone, adipose (fatty) tissue, or water. Obesity is defined as an excessive amount of adipose tissue.

Causes of Being Overweight and Obese

Essentially, being overweight and obese comes from an energy imbalance. The body needs a certain amount of energy (calories) from food to sustain basic life functions. Body weight is maintained when the number of calories eaten equals the number of calories the body expends, or burns. It's really basic math. When more calories are consumed than are burned, the energy balance is tipped toward weight gain, being overweight, and obesity.

The Risks Associated with Being Obese

Morbid obesity is associated with more than thirty illnesses and medical conditions, including:

- Type 2 diabetes
- Coronary heart disease
- Stroke
- Hypertension
- Cancer
- Asthma
- Osteoarthritis and joint degeneration
- Cirrhosis of the liver
- Venous stasis disease
- Infertility
- Gastroesophageal reflux disease (GERD)
- Chronic headaches
- Liver disease
- Sleep apnea
- Lower back pain
- Urinary incontinence

More importantly, obesity is associated with over 112,000 U.S. deaths each year. Obese individuals have a 10 to 50 percent increased risk of death compared to individuals of healthy weight.

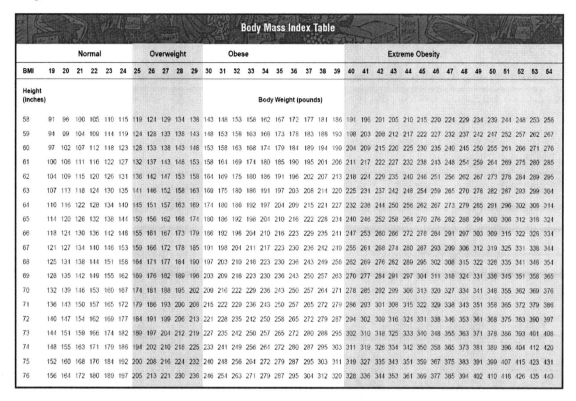

	Normal						Overweight					Obese										Extreme Obesity														
BMI	19	20	21	22	23	24	25	26	27	28	29	30	31	32	33	34	35	36	37	38	39	40	41	42	43	44	45	46	47	48	49	50	51	52	53	54
Height (inches)												Body Weight (pounds)																								
58	91	96	100	105	110	115	119	124	129	134	138	143	148	153	158	162	167	172	177	181	186	191	196	201	205	210	215	220	224	229	234	239	244	248	253	258
59	94	99	104	109	114	119	124	128	133	138	143	148	153	158	163	168	173	178	183	188	193	198	203	208	212	217	222	227	232	237	242	247	252	257	262	267
60	97	102	107	112	118	123	128	133	138	143	148	153	158	163	168	174	179	184	189	194	199	204	209	215	220	225	230	235	240	245	250	255	261	266	271	276
61	100	106	111	116	122	127	132	137	143	148	153	158	164	169	174	180	185	190	195	201	206	211	217	222	227	232	238	243	248	254	259	264	269	275	280	285
62	104	109	115	120	126	131	136	142	147	153	158	164	169	175	180	186	191	196	202	207	213	218	224	229	235	240	246	251	256	262	267	273	278	284	289	295
63	107	113	118	124	130	135	141	146	152	158	163	169	175	180	186	191	197	203	208	214	220	225	231	237	242	248	254	259	265	270	278	282	287	293	299	304
64	110	116	122	128	134	140	145	151	157	163	169	174	180	186	192	197	204	209	215	221	227	232	238	244	250	256	262	267	273	279	285	291	296	302	308	314
65	114	120	126	132	138	144	150	156	162	168	174	180	186	192	198	204	210	216	222	228	234	240	246	252	258	264	270	276	282	288	294	300	306	312	318	324
66	118	124	130	136	142	148	155	161	167	173	179	186	192	198	204	210	216	223	229	235	241	247	253	260	266	272	278	284	291	297	303	309	315	322	328	334
67	121	127	134	140	146	153	159	166	172	178	185	191	198	204	211	217	223	230	236	242	249	255	261	268	274	280	287	293	299	306	312	319	325	331	338	344
68	125	131	138	144	151	158	164	171	177	184	190	197	203	210	216	223	230	236	243	249	256	262	269	276	282	289	295	302	308	315	322	328	335	341	348	354
69	128	135	142	149	155	162	169	176	182	189	196	203	209	216	223	230	236	243	250	257	263	270	277	284	291	297	304	311	318	324	331	338	345	351	358	365
70	132	139	146	153	160	167	174	181	188	195	202	209	216	222	229	236	243	250	257	264	271	278	285	292	299	306	313	320	327	334	341	348	355	362	369	376
71	136	143	150	157	165	172	179	186	193	200	208	215	222	229	236	243	250	257	265	272	279	286	293	301	308	315	322	329	338	343	351	358	365	372	379	386
72	140	147	154	162	169	177	184	191	199	206	213	221	228	235	242	250	258	265	272	279	287	294	302	309	316	324	331	338	346	353	361	368	375	383	390	397
73	144	151	159	166	174	182	189	197	204	212	219	227	235	242	250	257	265	272	280	288	295	302	310	318	325	333	340	348	355	363	371	378	386	393	401	408
74	148	155	163	171	179	186	194	202	210	218	225	233	241	249	256	264	272	280	287	295	303	311	319	326	334	342	350	358	365	373	381	389	396	404	412	420
75	152	160	168	176	184	192	200	208	216	224	232	240	248	256	264	272	279	287	295	303	311	319	327	335	343	351	359	367	375	383	391	399	407	415	423	431
76	156	164	172	180	189	197	205	213	221	230	238	246	254	263	271	279	287	295	304	312	320	328	336	344	353	361	369	377	385	394	402	410	418	426	435	443

Use this table to determine if you may be a candidate for weight loss surgery.
Source: NIH, http://www.nhlbi.nih.gov/guidelines/obesity/bmi_tbl.pdf, August 2010

Who Should Consider Weight Loss Surgery?

According to the National Institute of Health (NIH), you may be a candidate for weight loss surgery if you are an adult with:

- a body mass index (BMI) of 40 or more (being about one hundred pounds overweight for men and eighty pounds for women) or a BMI between 35 and 39.9 and a serious obesity-related health problem(see BMI table above)

- acceptable operative risks
- an ability to participate in treatment and long-term follow-up
- an understanding of the operation and the lifestyle changes you will need to make

These guidelines for who should consider weight loss surgery also form the basis of most insurance coverage guidelines.

Like so many things in life, you need to consider the risks versus the benefits of having weight loss surgery. However, due to advances in medicine, weight loss surgery is recognized as both safe and effective.

According to the National Institute of Health, the risks of bariatric surgery have dropped dramatically and now are no greater than gallbladder or hip-replacement surgery. The risks are lower than the longer-term risk of dying from heart disease, diabetes, and other consequences of carrying more weight than a person's organs can tolerate. At thirty days post-surgery, researchers found the mortality rate among patients who underwent a Roux-en-Y gastric bypass or laparoscopic lap band to be 0.3 percent, and a total of 4.3 percent of patients had at least one major adverse outcome. An accompanying editorial stated the "surgery is safe, effective and affordable" because it can lower the number of doctor visits, medication use, and other medical expenses.

Among the most common weight loss surgeries, lap band surgery has the lowest risk. According to the manufacturer of the LAP-BAND® System, the mortality rate for lap bands is 0.05 percent, versus .5 percent for Roux-n-Y gastric bypass.

Special Considerations for Patients with Diabetes

There are new studies underway concerning weight loss surgery and diabetes. One study released in June 2009 by JAMA found that morbidly obese patients who have laparoscopic lap band surgery (LAGB) can expect sustained weight loss and an 83 percent improvement or remission of type 2 diabetes, with a significant reduction in hemoglobin (HbA1c) five years after surgery.

In January 2009, the American Diabetes Association's Standards of Medical Care in Diabetes added a section on bariatric surgery recommending that bariatric surgery should be considered for adults with a BMI of 35 kg/m2 and type 2 diabetes, especially if the diabetes is difficult to control with lifestyle and pharmacologic therapy.

Benefits of Bariatric Surgery

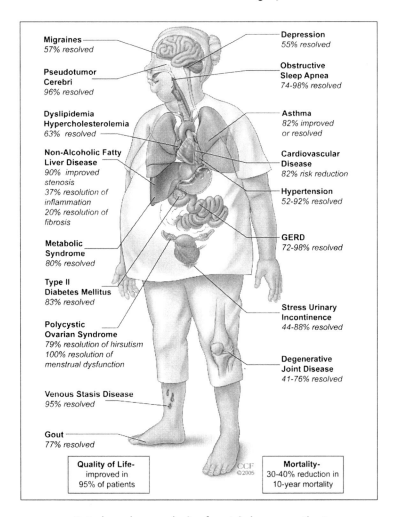

Migraines
57% resolved

Pseudotumor
Cerebri
96% resolved

Dyslipidemia
Hypercholesterolemia
63% resolved

Non-Alcoholic Fatty
Liver Disease
90% improved
stenosis
37% resolution of
inflammation
20% resolution of
fibrosis

Metabolic
Syndrome
80% resolved

Type II
Diabetes Mellitus
83% resolved

Polycystic
Ovarian Syndrome
79% resolution of hirsutism
100% resolution of
menstrual dysfunction

Venous Stasis Disease
95% resolved

Gout
77% resolved

Depression
55% resolved

Obstructive
Sleep Apnea
74-98% resolved

Asthma
82% improved
or resolved

Cardiovascular
Disease
82% risk reduction

Hypertension
52-92% resolved

GERD
72-98% resolved

Stress Urinary
Incontinence
44-88% resolved

Degenerative
Joint Disease
41-76% resolved

Quality of Life-
improved in
95% of patients

CCF
©2005

Mortality-
30-40% reduction in
10-year mortality

Data based on analysis of gastric bypass patients;
resolution of co-morbidities in lap band patients is similar.
Reprinted with permission of Cleveland Clinic.

Is Weight Loss Surgery the Easy Way Out?

I've spent a lot of time contemplating whether weight loss surgery is the easy way out. After talking with many people, professionals as well as patients, I have come to the conclusion that there are strong arguments for both sides.

Weight Loss Surgery Is the Easy Way Out

- *Some say it's easy because it is the only choice that makes sense for them. These are people who have failed multiple times over many years of dieting, people who may have other medical conditions that require them to lose weight in order to remain active, productive members of society.*
- *It has been compared to the "ease" with which a cancer patient chooses chemotherapy. While this may be a bit harsh, it makes the point. It's easy to choose something that may cure you over doing nothing and letting the disease take over.*
- *It provides hope where none existed for a significant population. Many of those who are exploring weight loss surgery have tried every diet out there, had some minimal success, but could not sustain that success. The possibility of achieving and maintaining a healthy weight provides a light at the end of a tunnel for those in the dark.*
- *It confirms that rather than a moral failing, obesity is a medical issue that can be addressed with a medical intervention. This is significant. The obese population has been discriminated against in every area of their life, and the recognition that medical intervention is necessary offers another ray of hope.*
- *It is easy because it works. This is true, but only at the beginning of the journey. Once the surgery starts working, the patient must learn the behaviors necessary to keep it working. Weight loss surgery is a tool. Screwdrivers work, but only if someone is on the other end of them turning the screw in the direction it needs to go.*
- *It is easy because patients, often for the first time in their lives, get the opportunity to physically feel full. The general population cannot begin to understand what it is like to finish a meal and be hungry again two minutes later. Weight loss surgery provides a "stop" that allows patients to recognize when they are done eating and to actually feel a sense of satiety.*

Weight Loss Surgery Is Not the Easy Way Out

Making a decision to have major surgery is not easy. Think about an obese person undergoing general anesthesia. This is not a simple decision. There are risks involved, and the benefits need to outweigh the risks for those who make that tough decision to go forward with surgery.

- *It is difficult to make the choice to not use food for comfort or reward. This is probably the first step to permanent lifestyle change that needs to be made.*
- *It is difficult because it requires permanent lifestyle changes in order to lose the weight and keep it off. The surgery is only a tool, and the patient is the one that chooses his or her food and chooses when and how much to exercise. It takes years to undo the years of poor choices that became regular behaviors.*
- *It is difficult because most weight loss surgery patients have to give up some foods permanently. There are some foods that are physically uncomfortable for weight loss surgery patients to eat and they may be among their favorite foods. Again, it's a hard choice to make and stay committed to.*
- *It is difficult to learn how to eat all over again—to take small bites, to chew food thoroughly, and to eat slowly. Our culture is one of on-the-go all the time. Weight loss surgery patients need to learn how to take time out for each meal and to pay attention to it so as to be able to avoid mindless eating or mindless overeating. The drive-through should become a thing of the past.*
- *It is difficult to suddenly change a lifetime of behaviors and stay committed to them. How long did it take to learn how to sit in front of the TV or computer instead of going for a walk? How long did it take before grabbing something on the way home became the expected meal. It will take years to make the new behaviors part of a standard routine that is as habitual as grabbing a coffee on the way to the office.*
- *It is difficult to learn the difference between fullness and satiety. We are hardwired to eat to fullness, but we have to learn to stop before we get that time-to-unbutton-the-pants feeling.*

Committing to a New Life

What surfaces here is that people who choose weight loss surgery as a means to an end, that end being a healthy, normal weight, have to commit themselves to a lifetime of behavior changes—food choices, portion sizes, exercise, etc.—in order to achieve their goals. Nothing about the decision to have surgery or to make those changes is easy. The remotely easy part of this process is the knowledge that there may finally be hope for those who have failed year after year at trying to achieve and maintain a normal weight with diet and exercise alone.

—Sandi

Become Familiar with Common Weight loss Surgeries

Why I Chose Lap Band

Back in 2005, I found it very hard to thoroughly research which surgery was best for me. The two most common procedures at the time that would be appropriate for me were the adjustable gastric band (the AGB or lap band) and Roux-en-Y gastric bypass (RYGB). I ordered every book I could find and read the binder the doctors gave me cover to cover. I found my way into the American Society for Metabolic and Bariatric Surgeons (ASMBS) website and printed out all the briefs from their 2005 meeting. I still couldn't decide which surgery to have. As the mother of two young children, I had difficulty justifying the risks of gastric bypass. But I was also scared based on what I was hearing that if I chose the lap band I wouldn't be as successful as a bypass patient. I was also scared that if I chose bypass I might die on the table or I'd be plagued with severe nutrition problems. It was hard for me to justify gastric bypass, but I was also more afraid of failing (again).

Once I was able to assemble enough information, I chose the lap band for three reasons:

- *Long-term success with the lap band. I kept going back to a slide presented at the informational seminar. Long-term results with the band are enduring and similar to those of gastric bypass patients at three years and beyond according to published studies.*
- *The lap band has the lowest risk profile.*
- *I'd met real people who had gotten great results from the procedure. I wanted what they had, and I found a doctor who I trusted and who believed I could be successful with a lap band.*

—Gloria

There are four types of operations that are commonly offered in the United States: adjustable gastric band (AGB) or lap band, Roux-en-Y gastric bypass (RYGB), biliopancreatic diversion with a duodenal switch (BPD-DS), and vertical sleeve gastrectomy (VSG). Each has its own benefits and risks. To select the option that is best for you, you and your physician should consider that operation's benefits and risks along with other factors, including your BMI, eating behaviors, obesity-related health conditions, and previous operations.

Adjustable Gastric Band
(the LAP-BAND® System, REALIZE® Band, and Others)[1]

The lap band works primarily by decreasing food intake. Food intake is limited by placing a small bracelet-like band around the top of the stomach to produce a small pouch about the size of a thumb. The outlet size is controlled by a circular balloon inside the band that can be inflated or deflated with saline solution to meet the needs of the patient. Long-term studies indicate that at three years and beyond, the weight loss with lap band is comparable to the Roux-en-Y gastric bypass.

Roux-en-Y Gastric Bypass

Gastric bypass (also known as the Roux-en-Y) is a combination procedure using both restrictive and malabsorptive elements, meaning that you absorb fewer nutrients and calories. It works by restricting food intake and by decreasing the absorption of food. The food intake is limited by a small pouch that is similar in size to the adjustable gastric band. In addition, absorption of food in the digestive tract is reduced by excluding most of the stomach, duodenum, and upper intestine from contact with food by routing food directly from the pouch into the small intestine.

With this surgery, first the stomach is stapled to make a smaller pouch. Then most of the stomach and part of the intestines are bypassed by attaching (usually stapling) a part of the intestine to the small stomach pouch. Gastric bypass is nonadjustable and has an increased risk of postoperative complications.

---

1 LAP-BAND° is a registered trademark of Allergan Inc. REALIZE° is a registered trademark of Ethicon Endo-Surgery, Inc.

Comparing LAP-BAND® System to Gastric Bypass

Source: Allergan, manufacturer of the LAP-BAND® System

LAP-BAND® System	Gastric Bypass
Procedure Differences The LAP-BAND® System requires no cutting, stapling, or removal of any part of your existing stomach, nor any intestinal rerouting.	In this procedure, cutting and stapling of stomach and bowel as well as rerouting of the intestine is required.
Adjustability Can be quickly, easily, and non-surgically adjusted to affect weight loss results — during a brief doctor's office visit.	To make any "adjustments" or to improve weight loss results from this procedure, additional surgery may be necessary.
Reversibility The LAP-BAND® System is reversible and, if necessary, can be removed — with the stomach usually returning to it's original shape.	Extremely difficult to reverse, requiring additional, complicated surgery — without guarantee of success.

LAP-BAND® System	Gastric Bypass
Results Long-term results (three to five years) with the LAP-BAND® System yield comparable results to the gastric bypass — without the associated risks of the more invasive bypass procedure.	May offer more rapid initial weight loss, but some patients with gastric bypass will regain some weight over time. After about three years, weight loss is comparable to the LAP-BAND® System.
Risks A less invasive operative procedure, the LAP-BAND® System also has a lower rate of operative complications. Since none of the intestine is removed or bypassed, there are low risks of problems absorbing necessary nutrients. You will not lose as much lean muscle mass and bone mass as with gastric bypass, which means you maintain more of the lean muscle mass you need to keep your metabolism working effectively. There is no risk of "Dumping Syndrome" since no part of the intestinal tract is bypassed with the LAP-BAND® System. Mortality rate: 0.05% Total complications: 9% Major complications: 0.2% Most common include: • Standard risks associated with major surgery • Nausea and vomiting • LAP-BAND® System slippage • Stoma obstruction The risk of short-term death following surgery is 10 times less compared to gastric bypass. For more safety information, visit www.lapband.com/en/learn_about_lapband/safety_information.	As stomach cutting, removal and stapling are involved in this procedure, gastric bypass can also have more operative complications. As this procedure "bypasses" a portion of your intestine, it may increase the risk for anemia, osteoporosis and other medical complications due to nutritional and vitamin deficiencies. In addition, you may lose more lean muscle mass than you will with LAP-BAND®. Risk of "Dumping Syndrome" — a condition that may occur when food is rapidly passed (dumped) from stomach to upper intestine. Symptoms may include cramps, nausea, speeding or slowing of the heart, etc. Mortality rate: 0.5% Total complications: 23% Major complications: 2% Most common include: • Standard risks associated with major surgery • Nausea and vomiting • Separation of stapled areas (major revisional surgery) • Leaks from staple lines (major revisional surgery) • Nutritional Gastric bypass has a higher risk of short-term death following surgery compared to LAP-BAND®.

Biliopancreatic Diversion with a Duodenal Switch

BPD-DS, usually referred to as a duodenal switch, is a complex bariatric operation that principally includes (1) removing a large portion of the stomach to promote smaller meal sizes, (2) rerouting food away from much of the small intestine to partially prevent absorption of food, and (3) rerouting bile and other digestive juices, which impairs digestion.

In removing a large portion of the stomach, a more tubular gastric sleeve (also known as a vertical sleeve gastrectomy, or VSG) is created.

The smaller stomach sleeve remains connected to a very short segment of the duodenum, which is then directly connected to a lower part of the small intestine. This operation leaves a small portion of the duodenum available for food and the absorption of some vitamins and minerals.

However, food that is eaten by the patient bypasses the majority of the duodenum. The distance between the stomach and colon is made much shorter after this operation, thus promoting malabsorption. BPD-DS produces significant weight loss. However, there is greater risk of long-term complications because of decreased absorption of food, vitamins, and minerals.

Vertical Sleeve Gastrectomy

Vertical Sleeve Gastrectomy (VSG) historically had been performed only as the first stage of BPD-DS (see above) in patients who may be at high risk for complications from more extensive types of surgery. These patients' high risk levels are due to body weight or medical conditions. However, more recent information indicates that some patients who undergo a VSG can actually lose significant weight with VSG alone and avoid a second procedure. It is not yet known how many patients who undergo VSG alone will need a second-stage procedure. A VSG operation restricts food intake and does not lead to decreased absorption of food. However, most of the stomach is removed, which may decrease production of a hormone called ghrelin. A decreased amount of ghrelin may reduce hunger more than other purely restrictive operations, such as gastric band. Since a portion of the stomach is removed the sleeve gastrectomy is permanent.

Are You a Candidate for Lap Band Surgery?

According to Allergan, the manufacturer of the LAP-BAND® System, you may be a candidate if:
- Your body mass index is at least 40, or
  - » your BMI is 35 or higher with one or more obesity-related health conditions.
  - » you are at least 100 pounds overweight.

- You are at least eighteen years old.

- You have been overweight for more than five years.

- Your serious weight loss attempts have had only short-term success.

- You are not currently suffering from any other disease that may have caused your excess weight.

- You are prepared to make major changes in your eating habits and lifestyle.

- You do not drink alcohol in excess.

- You are not currently pregnant. (Note: If you become pregnant after having this procedure, the band can be adjusted for the duration of your pregnancy.)

Adjustable gastric banding is less invasive than other weight loss surgeries, but it is still a surgical procedure and has risks involved. You must discuss all of the risks and benefits of your specific case with your doctor in order to make an informed decision.

Remember, the information provided in this book (including all text, graphics, and images) is for informational purposes only. It is not intended to be construed, nor should the reader construe it as, medical care or medical advice, and it is not a replacement for medical care given by physicians or trained medical personnel. Readers should always seek the advice of their physicians or other qualified healthcare providers when experiencing symptoms or health problems, or when investigating the possibility of treatment. The authors are patients, not physicians, and speak only of their personal experiences and about the information they have gathered over time. Please refer to the complete medical disclaimer at the beginning of this book.

Exercise 1: Finding Out if Weight Loss Surgery Is Right for You

Assess whether you are a candidate for weight loss surgery.

What is your BMI?

_____

What are your health problems that may be associated with obesity?
(These health problems are commonly referred to as co-morbidities.)

_____

_____

_____

_____

_____

_____

_____

_____

_____

_____

Do you meet NIH guidelines for weight loss surgery?

_____

If you do not meet NIH guidelines for weight loss surgery, do you still want to research weight loss surgery? If yes, why? (Be prepared to discuss these reasons with your doctor.)

_____

_____

_____

Which surgery are you most interested in and why?

_____

_____

_____

_____

_____

Useful Websites

For some of the most current and unbiased information on obesity and obesity surgery, you can also refer to these websites:

- http://www.asmbs.org (American Society for Bariatric and Metabolic Surgery)
- http://www.win.niddk.nih.gov (The Weight-control Information Network, or WIN, is an information service of the National Institute of Diabetes and Digestive and Kidney Diseases (NIDDK) and the National Institutes of Health (NIH).
- http://www.obesityaction.org (Obesity Action Coalition)
- http://www.bandedliving.com Banded Living is a community for lap band patients,

by lap band patients

- The manufacturers of the lap bands also have very informative sites where you can usually find their latest research and patient information:

  » http://www.lapband.com/en/home/ (Allergan, the manufacturer of the LAP-BAND system)

  » http://www.realize.com (Ethicon Endo Surgery Inc, a Johnson & Johnson company, manufacturer of the REALIZE band)

NOTES

_____
_____
_____
_____
_____
_____
_____
_____
_____
_____
_____
_____
_____
_____
_____
_____
_____
_____
_____
_____
_____
_____
_____
_____
_____
_____
_____
_____
_____
_____
_____

NOTES

NOTES

_____

_____

_____

_____

_____

_____

_____

_____

_____

_____

_____

_____

_____

_____

_____

_____

_____

_____

_____

_____

_____

_____

_____

_____

_____

_____

_____

_____

_____

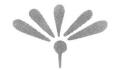

Peder's Story

My name is Peder. I am the father of three awesome young adults. I put everything I had into raising them but had forgotten all about me. After they all were in college I went to the doctor for my first physical in twenty-plus years. I got on the scale at my doctor's office and was too heavy for it. I was over four hundred pounds, a major blow to my self-esteem.

My doctor asked if I had ever considered bariatric surgery, since dieting was clearly not working. She sent me to see doctors over sixty miles away for a consultation. I am not a person who likes doctors; I pass out at the sight of a needle, so, as you can imagine I was very reluctant to have surgery.

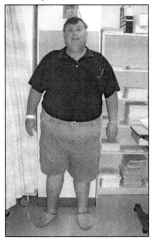

Peder before lap band surgery

Two years later, and still unable to be weighed at the doctor's office, I decided I had to do something. My doctor gave me a new list of surgeons this time and came up with a world-renowned surgeon right in my own backyard. So I made the appointment that changed my life. I went in for my first consultation and walked out of the office knowing that I found a surgeon I trusted. What a great group of doctors and techs; they made me feel great.

After getting surgery approved by my insurance company, I scheduled my lap band surgery for May 27, 2009. That is the day my life changed forever. I got on the scale at the hospital and it read 448.5 pounds, and I knew I had made the correct decision. Surgery turned out to be a breeze for me. I have no idea why I feared it so much.

I see the RN every month and have followed my surgeon's directions for one year. I now weigh 339 pounds. I am down over 100 pounds. The practice also uses successful patients as "angels" assigned to help me through tough times and to help answer any questions I have.

These patients are a true blessing. My angel and all of the office staff helped me through one of the toughest times of my life when my mother ended up in an ICU for over twenty days and is now in long-term rehab. I subconsciously remembered what they had been teaching me

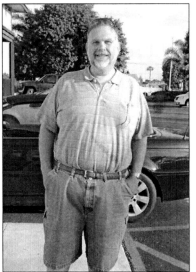

Peder transforming with lap band surgery

for ten months and lost another five pounds, instead of the ten I would have expected to gain while going through this difficult time. I have a great support team, so I am always around people that are on the same journey as I am—to live a happier, healthier, and longer life.

It has not been easy to change forty-nine years of bad habits, but with my lap band and my support system, it has been an enjoyable process. I hate medication almost as much as I hate needles, and I went from five medications per day to none!

I rode a bicycle for the first time in over seventeen years. I just got up on it and went. I love it, and now I walk and ride my bike and actually enjoy exercising every day. I lost 115 pounds in my first year and am still losing.

I now fit into booths at restaurants, I can move my body, I feel better, and I know I am much healthier.

I hope my story will be helpful to at least one person who is struggling to find the courage to have bariatric surgery and take control of their weight problem.

Step 2: Build Your Team

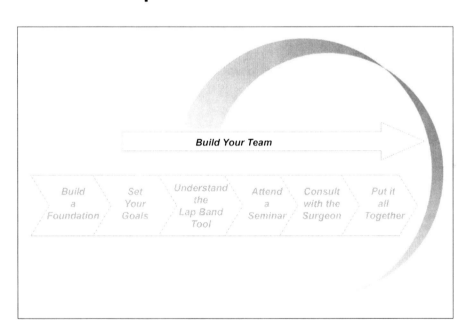

Objectives

The objectives of this step are to guide you to be able to:

- Understand who you need on your team and why
- Determine whether or not you have the support you need

Introduction

So why is it important to talk about teams? Like so many other things in life, there is no substitute for building the best team. Regardless of which lap band you choose, it is important to surround yourself with the right people to help you make the best informed decision and to support you on your journey. Building a team to support you on your journey is an ongoing process, one that is critical to your success. During the exploring phase, it is helpful to actively begin to put together your team. Your team will grow and change throughout the years.

Understand Who You Need on Your Team and Why

Loved Ones

A Partner on This Journey

> *I approached my husband about the idea of surgery. I wasn't expecting to get the support that I was looking for, but my husband surprised me. He said that if I was doing it for my health, I should look into it. He has been with me every step of the way. I don't know that I have the words to express how grateful I am for his unwavering support. I married a very special man. He has always proven to me that when times get tough, we get stronger together. I am so grateful to have him with me on this journey.*
>
> *—Gloria*

Do the most important people in your life know you are thinking about surgery? Do they support you? Will they be involved in the decision process? We've learned that it is important not to underestimate the impact of this life-changing decision on those closest to you. Be sure to include them in your research and discussions. If possible, bring them to seminars, support groups, and doctor appointments.

If you choose to go ahead with surgery, they may be worried. You'll be changing quickly, and that means a lot of change for those closest to you. The eating habits of everyone in your household may change as a by-product of your surgery. It's a lot easier for your loved ones to adapt to this change if they are part of the exploration process.

Exercise 2: Build Your Team—Loved Ones

List members in your immediate household. Answer the questions below for each family member.

_____

_____

_____

_____

_____

Do they know you are exploring surgery?

_____

_____

_____

_____

_____

Will they support your decision?

_____

_____

_____

_____

_____

What do you need from them?

_____

_____

_____

_____

_____

How will they be involved in the process?

_____

_____

_____

_____

_____

Primary Care Physician
Finding the Right Match

After working with the same internist for over twelve years—who had seen me through a lot—I moved to California and had to find a new primary care doctor. Given that my weight was my biggest health issue, I sought out the only primary care doctor who was also certified in bariatric medicine in my town. After working with him for about a year, I talked with him about getting weight loss surgery. After reviewing my records, he said that I had lost fifty pounds before and I could do it again. He was against surgery and didn't think it worked. I decided that I needed to find another doctor to see me through this journey, so I found a wonderful new doctor who was willing to learn about lap band surgery with me. I'll never forget a routine visit two years after getting my lap band when she walked into the exam room and exclaimed, "Look at you, you're a perfect specimen!"

—*Gloria*

Work closely with your primary care physician. He or she may encourage you to have lap band surgery or may discourage you. They may have a lot or very little experience with weight loss surgery. If you are in an HMO, you will probably need a referral from your primary care physician to see a specialist about weight loss surgery. It's okay if your doctor is early on in the learning curve; this is a new and growing area. Your doctor may be willing to learn with you, as obesity is the number two cause of preventable death in the United States. Your primary care physician is a critical member of your team.

Exercise 3: Your Doctor's Recommendations

If your primary care physician is recommending lap band surgery:

Does he or she recommend a surgeon? If so, who and why?

_____

_____

_____

_____

_____

Why is he or she recommending surgery (list reasons)?

_____

_____

Are there any specific concerns that your primary care physician has?

_____

_____

_____

_____

_____

If you are in an HMO, what are your plan's specific requirements from you and your primary doctor?

_____

_____

_____

_____

_____

If you are bringing the idea of lap band surgery to your primary care physician:

What has your doctor's experience been with other patients who have had lap band surgery?

_____

_____

_____

_____

_____

Does your doctor think you are a good candidate? Why or why not?

_____

_____

_____

_____

_____

Will your doctor support your decision to have surgery or not?

_____

_____

_____

_____

Bariatric Surgeon

The surgeon you pick will ultimately have your life in his or her hands in the operating room and can become your head coach for years to come. This needs to be a doctor you have researched and feel comfortable with. Do your homework. This is not your typical surgeon/patient relationship where something is broken, the surgeon fixes it, and you follow up once or twice and get on with your life. This needs to be a doctor that you want to see over and over again. Aftercare is essential.

There are many ways to find a lap band surgeon. You can be referred by:

- Your primary care physician (or other doctor)
- Other weight loss surgery patients
- Your insurance company (PPO or HMO)
- The manufacturers' websites (surgeon locators)
- Advertising

These sources can help you put together a list of doctors you may wish to see. You can then check their free informational seminar schedule.

Depending on your experiences, history, and insurance coverage, you may make your final decision about your surgeon at a different time in your journey. For example, if you have a family member who has had weight loss surgery, had a great experience, and the doctor is covered by your plan, you may already know who you want to use. On the other hand, you may be like Gloria, going through a long exploring process without any ties to a specific practice. Anywhere along this spectrum is fine. In addition, there may be geographic constraints and insurance requirements that direct you to specific practices.

Choose the exercises that relate to you, depending on your specific circumstances.

Exercise 4: Picking Your Bariatric Surgeon

Answer the following questions.

What surgeons are covered by your insurance in your area? (Skip if you are a cash-paying patient.)

_____

_____

_____

Do you have a preferred surgeon based on experience or recommendations?

_____

What do you know about the surgeons you are considering?

   »   Number of lap bands placed?

_____

   »   Affiliations with a Center of Excellence (COE)?

_____
_____
_____
_____
_____

   »   Word of mouth?

_____
_____
_____
_____
_____

Describe the surgeon's aftercare practice (including lap band adjustments or "fills," nutritional counseling, psychological counseling, exercise, lap band only support groups, and ease of reaching your doctor with questions in emergency situations)

_____
_____
_____
_____
_____
_____
_____
_____
_____
_____
_____
_____

How easy will it be to see this doctor or his or her staff four to twelve times over the first year?

_____

_____

_____

_____

What will your out-of-pocket costs be for each aftercare visit?

_____

How many surgeons are in the practice?

_____

Which surgeon will perform your surgery?

_____

_____

_____

_____

_____

Other Patients

There is tremendous value in learning from others who have lap bands. Our doctors often remind us that they don't have a band and that we need to learn from our peers. Find successful patients and learn from them. Research shows that those who participate in support networks achieve higher levels of success.

Friends and Colleagues

Beware of Well-Meaning Friends

I remember telling two of my closest friends that I was considering weight loss surgery. I was surprised by the lack of support I received. They said they didn't think I was fat enough to need surgery, but I wondered what they really thought as I sat uncomfortable in my black stretch-waist pants and my flowing top, courtesy of Lane Bryant. Just what is "fat enough"? Didn't they get that I met the guidelines for weight loss surgery? Didn't they get that I was miserable? Didn't they get that my kids' friends were going to make fun of them because their mother was fat! Didn't they get that I was afraid for my health? One of my closest friends really listened to me, but she still begged me not to have gastric bypass because she knew someone who had died from that surgery. That scared me.

—*Gloria*

It seems that a lot of people have an opinion about weight loss surgery. Some opinions are current but some are based on anecdotal experience that is twenty years old, often in the form of old "stomach stapling" horror stories. If you are exploring lap band surgery, it is important to think about who you are going to tell. There is no right or wrong answer here. It is a very personal decision. Think it through ahead of time because once you've told people, you cannot take it back.

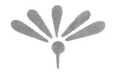

Betsy's Story

My battle with weight began in my *mother's* head. Painfully appearance-conscious, she placed a great deal of emphasis on how her children reflected upon her.

And there was *nothing* worse than being fat.

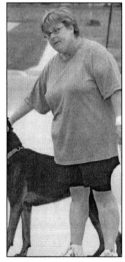

Betsy before lap band surgery

Looking back, I was a perfectly formed little girl. But I've been fat in the head my entire life. And because of a series of metabolism-killing diets inflicted on me beginning in elementary school, I developed a walking case of Obesity-Waiting-to-Happen.

It took a while for me to fulfill that prophecy. Though briefly chubby around puberty, I maintained a normal weight until I had kids. But I had to starve to stay there.

My weight skyrocketed during my first pregnancy. I managed to reach a normal weight after my second child—but not for long. Commercial diets failed me; despite meticulous attention to their rules, I gained. Group leaders looked at me askance, implied I was cheating. I felt as if I was again under the scrutiny of a disapproving mother—but I stuck with it—and added fifty pounds to my already bloated body.

In the early '90s, I worked in a Houston hospital where an earlier incarnation of gastric banding was performed. At the time, I swore I'd never have bariatric surgery—ever. But a chance encounter with a recent bandster made me rethink. One afternoon, the parents of one of my son's friends came to pick their son up. The woman mentioned her husband's weight loss over the preceding year. Curiosity piqued, I asked, "How did you do it?"

"I don't usually tell," he confessed, "but I have a gastric band."

Hm. Gastric band. The notion rattled around my brainpan for a good year as I continued to beat my head against the wall with ineffective dieting. Then one morning, I simply woke up knowing that gastric banding was my solution.

By noon that day, I'd registered for a seminar with BMI Surgery in Joliet, Illinois. My husband wasn't enthusiastic, so I invited him to join me. Dr. Brian Lahmann presented the basics of various bariatric surgeries: gastric banding, vertical sleeve gastrectomy, and Roux-en-Y gastric bypass. By the time he was done speaking, we were both very comfortable with what lay ahead.

My preop and operative course were textbook-smooth. I believe choosing the right surgeon made all the difference. Dr. Lahmann and his staff provide excellent patient education and aftercare—both of which are crucial to success. Also crucial for me have been (a) following a low-carb regimen, and (b) no-excuses exercise—every single day.

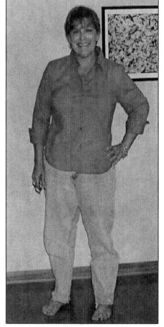

Betsy transforming with lap band surgery

The latter has been critical not only for promoting weight loss but getting me in touch with my body.

In just over eight months, I've gone from a BMI of 40 to 27.1. I'm about eleven pounds away from a normal BMI, and thirty-nine from my personal goal. I am thrilled with the loss I've experienced. But the internal changes catalyzed by my band have been far more remarkable. I no longer suffer from a killer case of *fat-in-the-head*.

This morning I got on the scale. It read 148.4. Nice! Good number—I was pleased.

Then, a while later, when I sat down to write, it hit me: *I've lost over one hundred pounds from my highest weight!*

Why is this significant? For my entire life, I have focused on reaching an elusive number on the scale. But this morning, I didn't immediately equate my weight with anything more than a nice loss for the work I've done over the past week. ***The number just doesn't matter all that much anymore!***

Yes, it's certainly a milestone. I'm thrilled to be 100.2 pounds down from my highest weight, 85 from my highest banded weight. But I'm far happier that the gray machine that sits on the floor of my bathroom no longer dictates my mood as it has, every day, since I was a very small child. If you had told me, 18 months ago, that the most valuable ring

I would ever receive would be made of flexible silicone, I would have thought you were crazy. But my gastric band was the best gift I've ever been given. It has transformed my body and my mind, shown me possibility, and allowed me to become who I was meant to be.

Exercise 5: Friends and Colleagues—Identifying Your Supporters and Naysayers

Answer the following questions.

Who will support you?

_____

_____

_____

_____

_____

_____

Who will judge you?

_____

_____

_____

_____

Who will sabotage you?

_____

_____

_____

_____

Who are you going to tell? (Remember, once you decide to tell someone, you can't take it back).

_____

_____

_____

_____

_____

_____

NOTES

_____
_____
_____
_____
_____
_____
_____
_____
_____
_____
_____
_____
_____
_____
_____
_____
_____
_____
_____
_____
_____
_____
_____
_____
_____
_____
_____
_____
_____
_____
_____
_____
_____
_____

NOTES

NOTES

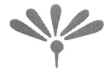

Chris's Story

I had my lap band surgery on December 20, 2004, only five months after first learning about the lap band.

When my cousin told my sister and me about her recent lap band, I was totally against any form of bariatric surgery. My sister, however, was interested in exploring lap band surgery, so while we were visiting other family, I was going online to do the research. The more I read, the more receptive I became. I decided to approach my primary care doctor, and he thought it might be a good option for me.

At the time, only a couple of clinics were performing lap band surgery in my area. I absolutely was not going to settle

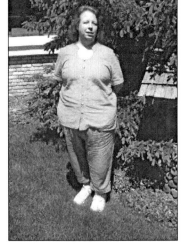

Chris before lap band surgery

for any bariatric surgery other than the lap band. I met with a surgeon in less than a month, and he explained how the lap band and RNY surgeries work. I was in the OR before I knew it, and my journey began.

My journey has been slow, but steady. My surgeon is very conservative about fills in the beginning. Initially, I needed to wrap my head around the new tool I had. Going into therapy was critical for me. It took me four and a half years to reach my personal goal of losing one hundred pounds, but I did it. I've

Chris transforming with lap band surgery

also had my first plastic surgery, which has given me further resolve to lose the next thirty-five pounds to reach my doctor's goal. Then I plan to go in for a tummy tuck.

Snags? There have only been a few. I had kidney stones four months post-op due to dehydration. My gallbladder was functioning at 12 percent (no stones) so I had surgery in October 2009. Five years after my surgery, I had a leaking port. My port has since been replaced, which was a relatively simple fix, and I'm now back on the losing track again. If these three things are the only complications in over five years, then I am not going to complain. I am determined that my band will be a tool I can use the rest of my life, as long as I maintain it.

Step 3: Set Your Goals

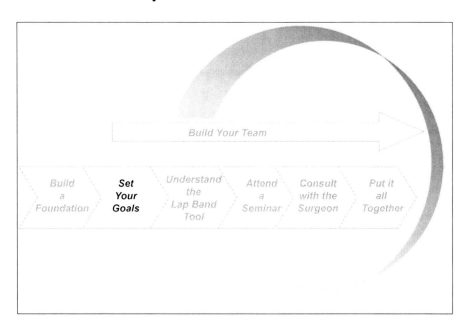

Objectives

The objectives of this step are to guide you to:

- Define what you want to achieve in terms of health, weight loss, and quality of life
- Assess whether or not your goals are realistic
- Redefine your goals with your eyes wide open

Introduction

If you've purchased this book, chances are that you've been on many diets. One thing we all have in common is that our way of losing weight hasn't worked. We'd all like a quick fix, but unfortunately there is none—at least not yet.

We each had very specific goals for our lap band surgery. At first, some of your goals may not be very realistic. Understanding what is realistic and what you can expect to achieve before you make your decision is critical to your success. The exercises below will help you set realistic expectations.

What Do You Want to Achieve in Terms of Health, Weight Loss, and Quality of Life?

Exercise 6: Define what you want to achieve when it comes to your health

List your current health problems.

_____

_____

_____

_____

_____

Which of the above are likely related to your weight? (Health problems related to your weight are referred to as co-morbidities.)

_____

_____

_____

_____

_____

Which health problems concern you most?

_____

_____

_____

_____

What is your family history concerning these medical conditions?

_____

_____

_____

What other health concerns do you have (current or future)?

_____

_____

_____

What health problems do you expect to resolve or improve with weight loss surgery?

_____

_____

_____

Assess Whether Your Health Goals Are Realistic

Enough Was Enough

I went to my primary care physician's office with yet another case of bronchitis. The nurse took my blood pressure and proceeded to quickly leave the room. In just a few moments the doctor came in with a strange look on her face. She took my BP again, then informed me that my blood pressure was high enough that she was concerned. At that point I was too frightened to even ask her what it was. I just felt as if I must be close to having a stroke if she came in to tell me this. She went on to explain that she would give me a pill and then monitor my blood pressure and let me leave when it went down a bit. I nodded agreement, put the pill under my tongue and proceeded to wait. What seemed like two lifetimes was probably about one half hour and finally, after taking my blood pressure two or three more times, I got to leave the office, prescription in hand. I was still too scared to ask for details, I was blindly following instructions, but had come to the conclusion that it was finally time to do something about my weight. I had had enough.

—Sandi

According to doctors at the Cleveland Clinic "Obesity-related diseases dramatically resolve or improve after bariatric surgery. No other medical or surgical intervention simultaneously treats as many disease processes as bariatric surgery does." Lap band surgery can improve your health, and quality of life. Take a look, once again, at the statistical results to help you set your goals.

Benefits of Bariatric Surgery

Migraines
57% resolved

Pseudotumor Cerebri
96% resolved

Dyslipidemia Hypercholesterolemia
63% resolved

Non-Alcoholic Fatty Liver Disease
90% improved stenosis
37% resolution of inflammation
20% resolution of fibrosis

Metabolic Syndrome
80% resolved

Type II Diabetes Mellitus
83% resolved

Polycystic Ovarian Syndrome
79% resolution of hirsutism
100% resolution of menstrual dysfunction

Venous Stasis Disease
95% resolved

Gout
77% resolved

Depression
55% resolved

Obstructive Sleep Apnea
74-98% resolved

Asthma
82% improved or resolved

Cardiovascular Disease
82% risk reduction

Hypertension
52-92% resolved

GERD
72-98% resolved

Stress Urinary Incontinence
44-88% resolved

Degenerative Joint Disease
41-76% resolved

Quality of Life- improved in 95% of patients

CCF ©2005

Mortality- 30-40% reduction in 10-year mortality

Data based on analysis of gastric bypass patients; resolution of comorbidities in lap band patients is similar. Reprinted with permission of Cleveland Clinic.

Redefine Your Health Goals
Exercise 7: Redefine what you want to achieve when it comes to your health

After reviewing the above facts and reading the realities of lap band outcomes, revise your definitions of what you want to achieve when it comes to your health after having lap band surgery. Remember not to set yourself up with unrealistic expectations.

Define what you want to achieve when it comes to your health

List your current health problems.

_____
_____
_____
_____
_____

List your current medications.

_____
_____
_____
_____
_____

Which of the above are likely related to your weight?

_____
_____
_____
_____
_____

Which health problems concern you the most?

_____
_____
_____
_____
_____

What is your family history with these medical conditions?

_____

_____

_____

_____

_____

What other health concerns do you have (current or future)?

_____

_____

_____

_____

What health problems do you expect to resolve or improve with weight loss surgery?

_____

_____

_____

_____

Exercise 8: Define what you want to achieve when it comes to weight loss

What do you weigh now?

_____

What is your goal weight after lap band surgery?

_____

Was there a time in your life when you were at a weight that felt comfortable? What was that weight? Why did you feel comfortable?

_____

_____

_____

_____

On the following pages, insert pictures of you over time, from childhood to present. Write below each picture the year and your approximate weight.

My Photos

My Photos

My Photos

Assess Whether Your Weight Loss Goals Are Realistic

Fact Check

It is important to know the statistics from lap band procedures to help you evaluate if this procedure is right for you. Below are some important facts to be aware of.

According to the manufacturer of the LAP-BAND® System, mean excess weight loss (EWL) achieved after surgery was

- 40 percent at twelve months
- 43 percent at twenty-four months
- 47 percent at thirty-six months

Weight Loss with the LAP-BAND® System is Comparable to Standard Gastric Bypass at 3 years and Beyond

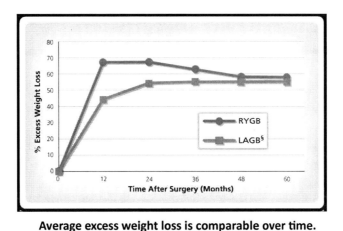

Average excess weight loss is comparable over time.
RYGB = Roux-en-Y gastric bypass
LAGB = Laparoscopic adjustable gastric banding
Laparoscopic adjustable gastric banding using the LAP-BAND® System and another adjustable gastric band. Comparison is based on pooled data from 43 peer-reviewed reports involving at least 100 patients at entry and providing at least 3 years of postoperative data. Data at the five-year point is reflective of N=176 patients for RYGB and N=640 patients for LAGB.
Individual results may vary.
Source: Allergan, manufacturer of the LAP-BAND®

"Results Not Typical"

Whenever I'm reading through weight loss tips and success stories, what always jumps out at me are the words that inevitably follow every story: "results not typical." So the truth is, my results for lap band surgery are not typical either, but what is typical? Expected results for me would have been to lose and maintain half of my excess weight. That is far better than the results I ever achieved with diet, exercise, drugs, and diet doctors.

I started my journey at 232 pounds. Early in my transformation, my surgeon told me that I should expect my weight loss to stall in the 170s. I could live with maintaining a weight in the 170s. It was a "happy weight" for me. I remembered when I had dieted to the 170s before, and I had felt good about the way I looked. I could wear normal-size clothing. I felt healthy. I wouldn't be the fat mom. And if I could just stop yo-yo dieting in the 170s, then I would have been good with that … but I'd always want more, because that is just who I am.

Needless to say, as my surgeon warned, I sailed pretty easily to the 170s, and then my weight loss stopped. I had a decision to make. Was I happy with where I was? Or was I willing to put in the work to get "results not typical"? I decided to go for it. Here is what I learned about how to achieve the "results not typical" with a band:

- *Journaling helped me find small changes in what I was eating, helping me increase protein and decrease calories. Journaling helped me be accountable to myself. Even today I still periodically journal.*
- *I always have a plan, or at least a plan B. I travel a lot and seem to have unlimited access to foods that can get me into trouble. I always have a supply of food with me to ensure my success. I'm not afraid to special order at restaurants or to ask a hotel to open the gym at 4:30 a.m. I have no excuses.*
- *Having a good support structure is critically important, forever. I am constantly building my team.*
- *I've come to terms with the fact that my weight loss is permanent. I am not going to fail again. I am not going to suddenly wake up fat again. I have a tool that helps with portion size, hunger, and satiety. As long as I use the tool, it will help me. Using my tool is based on behaviors, not intentions.*
- *Fills can still help. That's one of the features of the band that no other weight loss surgery offers.*
- *I stay close to my surgeon and his staff. I take advantage of the resources they offer.*
- *I pay it forward by helping others on their journeys. I am always learning, and it feels great!*

- *I work on my body image. It takes a long time to see my new body the way others see it. Liking what I see in the mirror helps me stay motivated. I am learning to say thank you when people compliment how I look. This was hard for me.*
- *I admit when I'm struggling and enlist help from my team.*
- *I periodically step up my exercise. The benefits of exercise are many-fold. Cardio burns calories; strength training builds muscle; more muscle burns more calories. Muscle is more compact than fat, so you lose inches. Exercise is good for my physical and mental health. Then there are those happy endorphins—I'm addicted. Exercise makes me feel good mentally and physically, which creates a wonderful cycle.*
- *I reward myself and take care of my body.*
- *I live my life. I do the things I've always avoided because I was too fat or embarrassed.*

So my results are not typical, but I strongly believe that if you define your goals, you can apply the lessons learned by others to achieve your goals for weight loss, health, and quality of life.

—Gloria

Redefine Your Goals

Exercise 9:

Redefine what you want to achieve when it comes to weight loss.

Review and revise your goal weight; what is a realistic goal weight?

_____

How do you honestly feel about your realistic goal? Will you be happy?

_____
_____
_____
_____
_____

How are you going to get there?

_____

_____

_____

_____

_____

Exercise 10:

Define what you want to achieve when it comes to your quality of life.

What can't you do because of your weight?

_____

_____

_____

_____

_____

List your feelings about how your weight affects your life and the lives of those you love (list the first five that come to mind).

_____

_____

_____

_____

_____

_____

_____

_____

_____

_____

Have you ever had an event that was a defining moment for you?

_____

_____

_____

_____

_____

_____

_____

_____

_____

_____

Here are some examples from our lives.

Breaking the Cycle

My mom died just a few days after her eighty-fourth birthday. I was with her day-in and day-out during her time in hospice care. I am grateful to everyone who gave me that time to be with her—my family, my employer, and my friends. It's strange: I was with my dad when he died, and I got to be with my mother when she died. Both my children are adopted (obesity is a known cause of infertility), and I was lucky enough to be in the delivery room for both of their births. It's the circle of life.

When the fog of my grief lifted, I decided once again that I was going to lose this weight, and break this cycle of obesity that runs in my family.

I had decided to start working out regularly again, since I was not traveling back and forth to see my mom. I started running on my treadmill. That was pretty hard on my joints with the weight I was carrying, but I was determined, and I pushed through the pain.

I went to see a podiatrist. He told me that I had a stress fracture, which made me feel pretty crappy. What I heard from that visit is, "What do you expect? You're fat. These things are going to happen ..."

—Gloria

Eyes Finally Wide Open

A defining moment came when I was vacationing in Aruba, weighing in at over four hundred pounds, driving everywhere, walking very little, eating massive amounts of food, and drinking high-calorie alcoholic drinks with umbrellas in them—because that's what you do on vacation. I love the ocean and am a certified scuba diver, but I realized I was too large to dive. The amount of lead it would take to keep me underwater would be more than I could possibly negotiate—probably in the neighborhood of thirty-five to forty pounds. So my husband and I went snorkeling instead. Off we went on this beautiful catamaran with about twenty-five other people for a fun afternoon in the sun, snorkeling by an old wreck. My husband geared up in mask, boots, fins, and snorkel and was in the water. I put on my boots and mask and then tried to get my fins on (which is next to impossible when you can't see your toes). I decided what the heck, I'll go in the water anyway—as big as I was I was still a strong swimmer. Snorkeling without fins definitely restricted the distance I could cover in the water. Then, to add insult to injury, hauling my fat butt back up onto the boat was a chore I was not prepared for. What was a really easy climb on the way down took me ten minutes back up, and I was huffing and puffing so much when I was back on board that the crew came over to make sure I was okay. Talk about humiliating!

—Sandi

Define Your Quality of Life Goals

Everyone's ideas of quality of life may be different. Some that we've heard before are to:

- Travel on a plane without a lap-belt extender
- Tie my own shoelaces
- Fit on the rides at an amusement park
- Play on the floor with my grandkids
- Set a good example for my children
- Meet the man or woman of my dreams, get married, and have a family
- Be treated with respect by strangers
- Be considered for a promotion
- Not be stereotyped as fat and lazy
- Say goodbye to plus-size stores
- Run a marathon
- Walk down the aisle at my child's wedding
- Use a normal size towel

I Choose Life!

When I set my goals, my ideal weight was 137 pounds—my realistic goal weight was 200 pounds. I wanted to be able to walk around Disneyland with my grandkids and fit on the rides with them. I also wanted to be able to do what most people take for granted—get down on the floor and play with them. I had been in a slow downward spiral, adding more weight and slowly killing myself in bits and pieces by restricting my ability to move around and enjoy physical activity. I wanted to fly to Tahiti and spend a week in an over-water bungalow snorkeling and diving. I wanted to be off all my meds and fit in an airplane seat, but I knew I would need to make some changes to get these things—changes that would require tough choices. I chose life!

—Sandi

Exercise 11: Quality of Life Goals:

List five things you would like to do after achieving your weight loss goals.

1. _____
2. _____
3. _____
4. _____
5. _____

Define Your Goals with Your Eyes Wide Open

Exercise 12: My Updated Goals

Now summarize your health, weight loss, and quality of life goals by listing them below.

Health

_____
_____
_____
_____
_____
_____
_____
_____
_____
_____

Weight Loss

_____
_____
_____
_____

Quality of Life

_____
_____
_____
_____
_____
_____
_____
_____
_____
_____

NOTES

_____
_____
_____
_____
_____
_____
_____
_____
_____
_____
_____
_____
_____
_____
_____
_____
_____
_____
_____
_____
_____
_____
_____
_____
_____
_____
_____
_____
_____
_____
_____
_____
_____
_____
_____
_____

NOTES

_____

_____

_____

_____

_____

_____

_____

_____

_____

_____

_____

_____

_____

_____

_____

_____

_____

_____

_____

_____

_____

_____

_____

_____

_____

_____

_____

_____

_____

_____

_____

_____

NOTES

_____

_____

_____

_____

_____

_____

_____

_____

_____

_____

_____

_____

_____

_____

_____

_____

_____

_____

_____

_____

_____

_____

_____

_____

_____

_____

_____

_____

_____

_____

_____

_____

_____

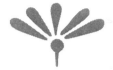

Gloria's Story

I have battled obesity for as long as I can remember. I vividly recall the pain and embarrassment of being weighed in my elementary school gym, praying that the school aide would not announce my weight for everyone to hear.

I started dieting at the age of ten. My days were defined as good or bad by what I ate and how my clothes fit. I have been on every diet you can think of. I took diet pills for years. I cannot remember a year when I didn't gain or lose at least forty or fifty pounds. My hunger never went away.

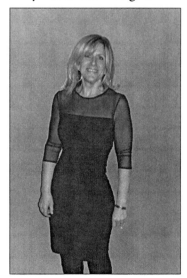

I was an overweight (okay—fat) child, an overweight teen, and an overweight adult. I spent my life yo-yoing. For me, dieting was like holding my breath: eventually, I had to come up for air. The irony is that except for my battle with weight, I've been successful at everything else I've ever attempted. I'm very fortunate. I have a great marriage, two wonderful children, true friends, and a successful career as an executive in Fortune 100 companies. But no matter how hard I tried, I could never take

Gloria before lap band surgery

off the weight and keep it off. I wasn't stupid, and I wasn't lazy. I was tired of doctors telling me that I needed to eat less and exercise more.

When I decided to get my band, I didn't tell anyone except for my husband and a few close friends. I was afraid I would

Gloria after lap band surgery

fail again. I was afraid of the stigma associated with being obese and "resorting" to weight loss surgery.

I have been maintaining a healthy, normal weight since 2007. I am now the fit girl at the gym. I am the active mom at school. I am the confident presenter in my business. And I am a more loving wife, because I no longer carry the burden of my weight on my body and in my heart. I am a different person today, and I love Banded Living. I feel confident that I will be able to maintain a healthy weight for the rest of my life.

Step 4: Understand the Lap Band Tool

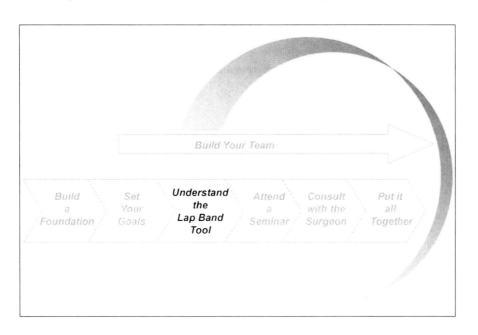

Objective

The objective of this step is to be able to understand why lap band surgery is different than all the diets you've been on by:

- Learning how the lap band works
- Learning what restriction is
- Learning how successful people use this tool
- Understanding the role of aftercare
- Understanding your eating habits and what needs to change with a band
- Understanding what you are willing to do to use the tool
- Recognizing what you are not willing to do

Introduction

"If you do what you've always done, you'll get what you've always gotten."

—*Anthony Robbins*[2]

All the diets we've been on work. The problem for us is that we haven't been able to stick with them, that is, until we got our lap bands. It is hard for someone without a band to understand what it feels like to have one. In this section we will try to give you a glimpse of what it is like to have a lap band.

You've already heard that the lap band is a tool. Like any tool, you need to learn how to use it and what to expect from it in order to get the results you want. Results with the band are enduring. Only one in twenty people are able to achieve long-term weight loss success with diet and exercise alone. For the other nineteen of us, weight loss surgery may be our best option.

We both did a lot of research on the surgeries. We chose the lap band because:

- It has a relatively low surgical risk
- There is a low level of serious complications
- Lap band surgery leaves your digestive system intact (no cutting or stapling of organs)
- There is no malabsorption
- It's easily reversible

---

2   Anthony Robbins cited in brainyquote.com, http://www.brainyquote.com/quotes/authors/t/tony_robbins.html.

- The weight comes off slowly and gradually; the average percentage of excess weight loss (EWL) of bypass and lap band surgery are about the same at five years

Different from Diets

I can't think of a commercial diet program I haven't been on. You name it, I've tried it. I was always a failure, losing twenty, fifty, seventy pounds for a while and then gaining it back. As long as I can remember, I fantasized about what it would be like to have a normal body. My band has helped me change my relationship with food. I am not always thinking about food or where my next fix will come from. From the doctors I've spoken to, we are still learning about why the band works. Taming an out-of-control appetite in humans is a very complex problem. We eat for all sorts of reasons; emotional eating is a big part of that equation. I can tell you that my band, used correctly, has helped me control my appetite. That's why it's different.

—Gloria

How the Band Works

The band works by restricting the amount of food you can comfortably eat and by helping you feel satisfied. What does that really mean? Let's start by understanding what a lap band looks like and how it is placed.

Stomach with LAP-BAND®

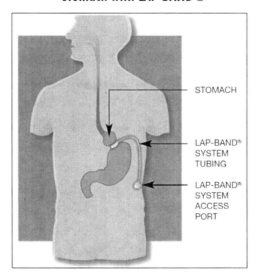

© Allergan, Inc.

The lap band is a silicone ring with an inflatable inner tube. It is placed around the upper portion of the stomach. Food enters the upper portion of the stomach, passes slowly through the area where the lap band is, and enters the lower stomach; picture sand going through an hourglass. Once food enters the lower portion of your stomach, normal digestion takes over from there. With this picture in mind, you can understand how the band helps you control volume.

If you talk with other patients, you will hear that the band helps with the feeling of being satisfied, of "having enough." The medical community is working to understand just how and why the lap band works to control hunger and satiety. Regardless, the band helps with real hunger. The band does not make emotional hunger go away. Emotional hunger comes from a different place, which the band will not help you with. It's important to recognize this.

With our lap bands, we are finally able to follow all the wonderful weight loss advice available. It feels great to find success with being able to control hunger issues and be in touch with our bodies and true hunger signals.

Reality Check

> *I had forgotten how much my band helped with satiety. After one and a half years, I began to take a normal appetite for granted … then I had a lesson in what life was like before my band.*
>
> *After the holidays, I decided my band was tighter than I liked and asked to have a small amount of fluid removed. The next day, I was ravenous. I feared that I might have a leak in my lap band system (an uncommon problem that is easily fixed). I called my doctor in a panic; he saw me right away. My doctor tried to remove the fluid from my band, but only a small amount came out. He gave me more fluid and repeated the process a few times over the course of a week, before concluding that my port probably did have a leak. I had my port and the fluid in the system replaced. Thank goodness the feeling of satiety returned. This was a clear reminder to me of how effective my band was at giving me a sense of satisfaction.*
>
> —*Gloria*

Learning about Restriction

You'll hear lap band patients talk about restriction. Restriction refers to how tight or how loose the band is. Remember, we said that the band is placed around the upper portion of the stomach. Restriction refers to the size of the opening between the upper and lower pouch and the sensation you feel based on the size of that opening.

Fill 'Er Up!

One of the greatest features of the band is that it is adjustable. The size of the opening between the upper and lower portions of your stomach can be made smaller or larger by having fluid added or removed. This has a direct impact on the amount of solid food you can eat comfortably in one twenty- to thirty-minute sitting and how satisfied you will feel from that meal.

From a patient's perspective, it can seem like both an art and a science to get your fill just right. This can require patience, but it will happen if you learn to listen to your body and work with your doctor. Many patients feel "unbanded" soon after surgery. This is common and just means you are healing and may benefit from a fill at your next office visit.

Don't Underestimate the Adjustable Nature of the Band

Adding saline tightens the band around your stomach, while removing saline loosens the band. We wasted a lot of time on message boards trying to figure out what the "right" fill should be. Nobody can tell you how many fills you will need to have to find your sweet spot because everyone is different. Gloria was one of those people who felt "unbanded" until she got to a good fill level. It took many fills to get to the right place where the satisfied feeling was reached with a small amount of food. Sandi, on the other hand, didn't need a fill her entire first year and still lost over a hundred pounds. And we both have the same size bands!

So the point is there is no magic number. The ideal fill is the level where you are satisfied with three small meals each day and you are not hungry between meals.

Lots of people worry about what a fill will feel like. It is not a big deal. If you can handle a needle stick, that's all there is. If you are sensitive, you can get a local anesthetic, but many people say the anesthetic needle hurts more than the needle used for the fill.

If you don't have a band, it is hard to understand the benefit of the adjustable nature of the band. Just when you think controlling your eating is getting hard, a little bit of tightening may be just what the doctor orders to get your weight loss going again. No other weight loss surgery is adjustable.

Knowing When It's Time for a Fill

The first year living with a band was an amazing experience for me. I saw my surgeon every four weeks to check my weight, my blood pressure, and my eating habits. I journaled religiously, recording every morsel that entered my mouth, every drop of liquid, and the nutrition content for all of it. Month after month, I hopped on the scale and was pleasantly rewarded with continued weight loss. I knew I had a band. My hunger between meals was pretty much gone, and I was satisfied with small portions at meals. But notice, I never said I was full. This is probably the most important distinction to understand and the most difficult to really get. As long as I was no longer hungry when I finished the portion I put on my plate, I was done. This was great because I was not hungry between meals either. Or, if I thought I was, I would have water or tea and suddenly wouldn't feel what I had interpreted as hunger pangs, but which were really thirst.

Month after month, just the lap band as it was installed produced consistent weight loss for me with no fills and no hunger. It was great. Then one day I was feeling hungry between meals. Really hungry. Water, iced tea, hot tea, nothing took care of it. It was scary. Fortunately, I had an appointment coming up the next week, so I white knuckled my way through it and made sure I didn't do anything differently. I checked my journal, making sure I was eating and drinking the same as before, and I was. The experience taught me how to know when it was time for a fill.

—Sandi

Rules of the Band

The manufacturers of the lap bands have their rules or tips published on their websites. What I learned from my fellow members of the Banded Living community is that (1) a lot of us don't like rules because we've tried them before and, frankly, they didn't work as a way of life, and (2) we are all different, and we need to work hard to find what works for ourselves.

So here I am, in my fifth year of having a lap band. I am maintaining a normal, healthy weight and am in the best shape of my life. I devote a lot of time and energy to helping others. I mentor lots of folks, some of whom are frustrated or struggling and trying to figure out how to get the most out of their tool.

My doctor, my head coach on this journey, reminds me over and over again, that the lap band is a tool and that I need to work with it. I shouldn't expect it to do anything, just like a screwdriver can't remove a screw unless I turn it. I have to work with it to get the results I want — and for me that was more than the average 50 percent excess weight loss. My band helps me with portion control, controls my hunger, and leaves me with a feeling of satiety when I use it.

Now, I'm not saying that I use my tool perfectly all of the time. What I am saying is that I've learned how to use my lap band to get great results and to keep myself in the same (small) pair of jeans for over two years. When I don't use my tool correctly, I gain a few pounds, but I know how to go back to basics and keep my weight within a normal, healthy range.

—Gloria

How Successful Patients Use Their Tool (Our Version of the Rules)

Here are the ten things that Sandi and Gloria have learned, as successful lap band patients, about how to use this tool.

1. **We stay close to our surgeon** and his staff. We have a whole team of people to help us on our journey. It starts with our surgeon, who acts as our coach. We also surround ourselves with other successful members of the Banded Living community.
2. We **don't drink with meals**. It prevents the band from working properly.
3. We make sure we get enough **protein** every day.
4. We eat good, **quality meals**, and we **don't graze**. We do best when we eat for twenty to thirty minutes and then leave the table.
5. We **don't drink our calories**. A properly adjusted band helps with portion control but only if we are eating solid foods. It doesn't restrict ice cream, a high-calorie frappuccino, or a frozen margarita.
6. We've learned to take **small bites and chew**, chew, chew. We also use small plates.
7. We've **learned what foods are difficult** for each of us and stay away from them. We have lots of great choices. We've learned to dine and enjoy food again.
8. We **always have a plan** for how we are going to use this tool. We don't give excuses.
9. We **journal when we need to**. We journaled consistently during our first years of banded living. When we wander off track or gain a few pounds, we go back to basics and journal for a while. It helps keep us in our target weight range by holding us accountable to ourselves.
10. We **make ourselves a priority**. We take care of our health, eat right, exercise, take our vitamins, and live life to the fullest!

Why is it so important that we don't drink with meals?

Picture a funnel. Pour liquid through the funnel and what happens? It flows right through. Your band works in a similar way. Liquids will go right through the narrow opening. High-calorie liquids will go through your band and directly to the places you least want it: your waist and hips!

Now picture pouring thick oatmeal through that funnel. The funnel eventually becomes full. That is the effect you want with your band.

Now picture what would happen if you watered down the oatmeal. It would flow through much faster. That is what happens when you drink with your meal when you have a band.

Protein

Protein is the most important nutrient for you to focus on. You should eat your protein first, then your vegetables, fruits, starches, and grains. You will work with your doctor to determine how much protein you need to have each day to feel satisfied, have energy, and maintain muscle mass. We generally hear a minimum of sixty to eighty grams of protein per day. (This is something you should discuss with your doctor or nutritionist; what is right for a five-foot-four woman is not what is right for a six-foot-two man).

When you are banded, it is helpful to keep track of how much protein you are eating. To give you perspective, one large egg has six grams of protein; three ounces of cooked chicken has twenty-six grams of protein; three ounces of canned tuna has twenty-one grams of protein; a half cup of cooked lentils has nine grams of protein. It is really important to understand the foods you like and where your sources of protein will come from. There are many websites that will help you find this out. One we use frequently is calorieking.com. Fitday.com is another popular site. Find one you like and use it, or get a book or an app for your PDA.

Eating with a Lap Band

Your daily nutrition should come from well-planned meals of quality solid foods. You will work with your doctor and his or her staff to help plan your meals.

The lap band works with solid foods. The band limits the amount of solid food you can comfortably eat in one twenty- to thirty-minute sitting. Most properly adjusted band patients say they can comfortably eat a half cup to one and a half cups of solid food with a properly adjusted band, but this varies from person to person. That may mean a half cup of chicken and a half cup to one cup of vegetables.

The band works by helping you feel satisfied after eating a small meal and by helping you control portion size. Stop at the first sign of feeling full. Do not linger at the table after the meal. You need to learn to slow down and chew well. The band will help you slow down and will remind you if you haven't chewed your food thoroughly because the food will feel as though it is stuck and will be uncomfortable.

If you are going to get the most from this tool, you must always have a plan for what you are going to eat. That may mean bringing your lunch to work, cooking for the week during the weekend, calling ahead to restaurants, or always carrying an emergency meal with you. Limit the amount of fat you use to prepare your food. Be aware of what is in the condiments you choose. Avoid high-calorie condiments.

You will hear different opinions about snacks. The best advice we've heard is to first master three meals a day and give up grazing. As lap band patients, we need to relearn what real hunger is, what it feels like to be satisfied after a meal, and how to construct high-quality meals every day.

If you do include snacks into your meal plan, a snack should be no more than one hundred calories, and it should contain protein (e.g., a slice of turkey wrapped around a pickle spear). Make sure the snack is scheduled into your day and that you are staying within your daily calories. However, some practices discourage tracking calories. Always follow your doctor's instructions.

Some Foods May Be Difficult to Eat After Having Lap Band Surgery

One of the most common questions we get is, "Are there any foods I will not be able to eat after surgery?" Most are relieved to hear that you can eat a wide variety of the foods you love with a lap band. However, there are some foods that banded people have trouble eating, such as:

- Bread
- Rice
- Pasta
- Steaks and chops
- Raw, fibrous fruits and vegetables

However, it's important to remember that we are all different and often have different reactions to which foods are easier to handle than others. Unfortunately, there is no way to predict which foods you will struggle with prior to surgery.

Understand the Role of Aftercare

Aftercare is critically important. How you set up and how you use your support team will help influence how successful you are with your new tool.

While each practice is different, the most successful patients visit their surgical practice between six and twelve times during their first year, at least once per quarter the second year, and at agreed to intervals thereafter. Your surgeon should be someone you believe can help you achieve your goals. You need to trust them and their staff, be willing to show up when you've fallen off the wagon, and fit those regular visits into your schedule. Sometimes you may need an adjustment or a fill, or sometimes you may need education.

Other patients are a great source of learning and support. You should plan to participate in a support community either in-person or online. Seek out the most experienced patients you can find, ones who've achieved what you hope to achieve and learn from them. Once you're well on your way, you may find it very fulfilling to help others.

My Angel

When I first met Sandi, she was just another patient from my surgeon's practice. I met her at a support group meeting. She impressed me immediately with her success, her knowledge, and, most of all, her deep caring and empathy. She soon became my angel, and I feel so incredibly fortunate to have her in my life. What I didn't know when I first met Sandi was that she would be there to hold my hand and teach me every step of the way on this banded living journey. In my fifth year, she's still there for me, and she's also one of my dearest friends. I doubt I would have been this successful without her; she taught me so much.
—Gloria

You may also want to see a nutritionist. Your doctor may have nutritionists on staff, or you may seek one out your own. If you do go out on your own, find a nutritionist experienced in helping lap band patients. A nutritionist with specialized band experience can help you make sure you enjoy what you are eating while also optimizing how you use your lap band.

Many lap band patients find that exercise helps in more ways than just burning calories and building muscle. Exercise can be a great stress reducer and can elevate endorphins, ultimately increasing energy levels. This can have many positive effects on your overall mood, self-esteem, and emotional well-being.

Giving Up Bad Habits

Habits are hard to break, but your post-op period is a great time to break them. One of the gifts of the post-op period is that most people have very little appetite. It is a strange and wonderful feeling for those of us who've struggled with hunger.

Habits you may need to give up are:

- Grazing—Grazing throughout the day counteracts how your lap band works. You need to eat high-quality meals to give yourself a chance to feel satisfied. If you continue to graze, you are not giving your tool a chance to do its magic. The good news is that you can use your recovery period to help break old habits.

- Nighttime eating—You've always known nighttime eating is bad for people trying to lose weight because it's a form of mindless eating. This holds true for band patients as well. Now is the time to create new eating habits and use your band to help you break this bad habit. If you must have something at night, follow the one-hundred-calorie snack rule.

- Eating in front of the television or eating while driving—Mindless eating has no place in your life. All studies show that people who consume food while distracted eat more. You owe it to yourself to learn to enjoy your food.

It took me about one and a half years, but I actually now really taste my food and enjoy what I eat. Eating has actually become more pleasurable.

—Sandi

- Bingeing—Bingeing and the lap band don't mix. The good news is that if you have a properly adjusted band, you physically will not be able to eat several slices of pizza, half the birthday cake left over from last night, or an entire bag of chips!

I'm On My Way

My doctor told me to schedule my post-op appointment four to six weeks after surgery, so of course I scheduled my appointment at the four-week mark—the sooner the better, I figured. I wanted to get out of the recovering phase and into the weight loss phase as quickly as possible. I still had a lot of old weight loss habits to break—it would be years until I finally realized that slow and steady wins this race. After all my years of dieting, all I wanted was to start losing as quickly as possible.

The day my post-op appointment arrived, I was already down nineteen pounds since my surgery. I knew I had begun losing weight on the post-op diet, but how much weight I had lost shocked me. I was thrilled! At the same time, I had to come to terms with the fact that I clearly didn't have a handle on just how much I had been eating. If I could lose that much weight in four weeks, I could no longer blame my slow metabolism for my life-long struggle with my weight.

After my physical exam, my doctor, who I really began to like and trust, began the first of many "mind adjustments." I totally underestimated the importance of this doctor-patient relationship. Over time, my surgeon worked on my head more than he ever worked on my body. He gave me a very direct lesson on learning to eat again. If I went back to my old eating habits, if I didn't work to learn to use my new tool, if I didn't come into the office regularly and attend support groups, I wouldn't have gotten the results I wanted—plain and simple.

Leaving the office on that day, I was thrilled. I was on my way!

—Gloria

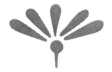

Chaz's Story

What can I say…my life had spun out of control somehow. How could this happen to me? I wish I knew. But in retrospect I think I can tell you there were a number of contributing factors.

I had battled my weight all of my life…from childhood until I was about nineteen years old. I was always teased, taunted, and picked on as a kid. It hurt, and I had no friends. At nineteen years old I decided that I had enough and was going to change my life. I would not turn twenty-one and be fat any longer. I had been on multiple diets from childhood, including diet pills. But I saw my life slipping away. I knew I did not have the kind of life other people had. So at twenty-one, by literally starving myself, and the help of amphetamine pills, I took off about 120 pounds and turned from the proverbial ugly duckling into the virtual swan. I was even discovered and approached to do fashion modeling and advertising. I was suddenly popular, and was pursuing my dream of being a singer and actor. It was like a dream come true. The only problem was…I wasn't happy.

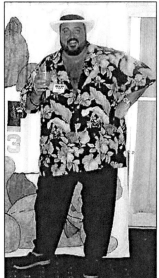

Chaz before lap band surgery

My head had not had a chance to catch up to my new body and the attention I was getting from everywhere. I didn't know how to respond appropriately to all the new changes in my life. As a result, some old insecurities and self destructive behaviors started to creep slowly back into my life. After a few years I started to pack on the pounds again. Like so many others, I tried every diet, weight loss programs, diet drugs, and every fad known to mankind in order to lose and hopefully maintain my weight. But this time it was to no avail. It was too late. The die was cast.

And I ended up gaining all the weight I had lost…plus another 100-plus pounds. I became depressed, sullen, and increasingly isolated. Previous to that time despite my weight issues I had always had a happy and positive outlook on life. I had turned from a positive thinking individual into someone who hid from the world, and had to secretly go weigh myself on a cargo scale at an airline where a friend of mine worked…because traditional scales couldn't hold me. It was humiliating.

Then things really began to spiral out of control. I was fired from an entertainment job for the very first time in my life because I had basically eaten myself out of the position. I was no longer attractive enough. Financial problems ensued. Then my younger brother died very suddenly, relationships went sour, and to top it all off, my wonderful mother, the light in my life, suffered a couple of debilitating strokes. I had to make the choice to give up my career, sell my home, leaving everything that was familiar to me, and at forty-eight years old move to Florida to become a full time caregiver to my elderly mother. I had no idea what I was in for.

I had always promised my mom that I would never put her in a nursing facility as long as I was physically able to care for her. But when I moved in to care for her I found out in short order that at 435 pounds, plus the kind of physical problems and co-morbidities I was experiencing, that I was not going to be able to fulfill that promise. THIS was *my* moment of truth. That is when I knew that without some kind of surgical intervention I was going to die and leave my dear and vulnerable mother alone. I simply could not allow that to happen.

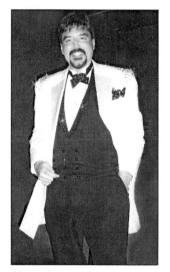

I had been checking into weight loss surgery for some time, and I somehow just knew that gastric banding was the right choice for me. I realized that it was a tool, and not the easy way out that some people would like to paint it as. And frankly, I was not the success story I wanted to be in the beginning. I was not the most compliant patient at first. But I persevered. And miraculously the weight started coming off…and STAYING off…for the first time in my life. And just as miraculously, my health, confidence, and self esteem began to return again after nearly twenty years. It took losing

Chaz after lap band surgery

215 pounds to finally rediscover the old me again. I was a new person, a more pleasant person to be around, and after almost eight years of caring for my mom I was gratefully able to fulfill my commitment to stay with her and hold her in my arms till her last breath.

Since then life has only gotten better for me. I am in a wonderful, healthy, committed relationship. I was able to start entertaining again. And I even developed a whole new career when my very own bariatric surgeon, Dr. Tiffany Jessee, asked me to come and work for her in her practice. This is something I would have never even dreamed possible only a few short years ago. Life is good!

As I see every new patient come into our office, I identify with each and every one of them and what they have gone through. There is an instant bond when they know my story, and I consider it a privilege and blessing to help guide and mentor them through their weight loss journey.

In September of 2010 I was also extremely proud to be among twelve people chosen from across the United States to go to Capitol Hill and speak to members of Congress and the media on the growing epidemic of obesity, as well as prevention and treatment. I remain an advocate and will work tirelessly to help be a voice for those who have lost theirs. I cannot think of a better or more appropriate legacy. My life has completely changed...all for the better as a result of bariatric surgery. It has been an incredible journey, and I would do it again in a heartbeat!

Understand Your Eating Habits and What Can Change with a Lap Band

Exercise 13: List the Diet Programs You've Been On

_____

_____

_____

_____

Which worked best for you and why?

_____

_____

_____

_____

_____

Which were least successful and why?

_____

_____

_____

Exercise 14: Identify Your Eating Patterns

Are you a volume eater?

_____

Are you a sweets eater?

_____

Are you a nighttime eater?

_____

Do you binge-eat (try to be honest with yourself)?

_____

_____

_____

Are you a grazer?

_____

How many meals per day do you eat?

_____

Which meals do you skip?

_____

_____

_____

_____

_____

Exercise 15: Keep a Food Journal for One Week

The purpose of this journal is *not* to eat well. The purpose is to have a realistic view of what you like to eat, when you eat, and where you eat. It's also good to have an idea of how much you eat on a typical day. It is hard to fix something if you don't know what is broken. This can help you identify where your problem areas are.

7-Day Food Journal

Day 1:

Time/Place   Food/Estimated Portion Size

Sample Entry:

7:30 am/car   *Egg McMuffin—1 sandwich (1 english muffin, 1 fried egg,*
                                    1 slice American cheese, 1 slice Canadian-style bacon, smear
                                    of liquid margarine)

                                    12 oz. (small) McCaffe Mocha (with sugar, whipped cream
                                    & chocolate syrup)

_____   _____
_____   _____
_____   _____
_____   _____
_____   _____
_____   _____
_____   _____
_____   _____
_____   _____
_____   _____
_____   _____
_____   _____
_____   _____
_____   _____
_____   _____
_____   _____
_____   _____
_____   _____
_____   _____

7-Day Food Journal

Day 2:

Time/Place	Food/Estimated Portion Size

7-Day Food Journal

Day 3:

Time/Place   Food/Estimated Portion Size

_____   _____
_____   _____
_____   _____
_____   _____
_____   _____
_____   _____
_____   _____
_____   _____
_____   _____
_____   _____
_____   _____
_____   _____
_____   _____
_____   _____
_____   _____
_____   _____
_____   _____
_____   _____
_____   _____
_____   _____
_____   _____
_____   _____
_____   _____
_____   _____
_____   _____

7-Day Food Journal

Day 4:

Time/Place   Food/Estimated Portion Size

_____   _____
_____   _____
_____   _____
_____   _____
_____   _____
_____   _____
_____   _____
_____   _____
_____   _____
_____   _____
_____   _____
_____   _____
_____   _____
_____   _____
_____   _____
_____   _____
_____   _____
_____   _____
_____   _____
_____   _____
_____   _____
_____   _____
_____   _____
_____   _____
_____   _____

7-Day Food Journal

Day 5:

Time/Place   Food/Estimated Portion Size

_____   _____
_____   _____
_____   _____
_____   _____
_____   _____
_____   _____
_____   _____
_____   _____
_____   _____
_____   _____
_____   _____
_____   _____
_____   _____
_____   _____
_____   _____
_____   _____
_____   _____
_____   _____
_____   _____
_____   _____
_____   _____
_____   _____
_____   _____
_____   _____

7-Day Food Journal

Day 6:

Time/Place   Food/Estimated Portion Size

_____   _____
_____   _____
_____   _____
_____   _____
_____   _____
_____   _____
_____   _____
_____   _____
_____   _____
_____   _____
_____   _____
_____   _____
_____   _____
_____   _____
_____   _____
_____   _____
_____   _____
_____   _____
_____   _____
_____   _____
_____   _____
_____   _____

7-Day Food Journal

Day 7:

Time/Place   Food/Estimated Portion Size

_____   _____

_____   _____

_____   _____

_____   _____

_____   _____

_____   _____

_____   _____

_____   _____

_____   _____

_____   _____

_____   _____

_____   _____

_____   _____

_____   _____

_____   _____

_____   _____

_____   _____

_____   _____

_____   _____

_____   _____

_____   _____

_____   _____

_____   _____

Exercise 16: Investigate the Nutritional Content of Your Favorite Foods

List ten solid foods that are a regular part of your normal diet. Look up the portion size, calories, and grams of protein in those foods. The purpose of this exercise is to be aware of the nutritional content of the foods you normally eat. Unless the food is fried, or exceptionally high in calories, many of these foods will probably be a part of your life after your lap band surgery. You need to know how they affect your diet.

	Food	Portion Size	Calories	Protein Grams
1.				
2.				
3.				
4.				
5.				
6.				
7.				
8.				
9.				
10.				

Exercise 17: Internalizing How the Tool Works

If you're reading this, you probably know that the traditional ways of losing weight and keeping it off don't work for you. The real question is: Can you use this tool to lose the weight you need to lose and keep it off? Try to be honest with yourself.

Rate each item below and on the following page on a scale of 1 to 5 (1 being the easiest, 5 being most difficult) based on how hard you think it will be for you to comply.

1. You can stay close to your surgeon and his staff: _____

2. You don't drink with meals: _____

3. You make sure you get enough protein: _____

4. You eat high-quality meals: _____

5. You don't graze: _____

6. You don't drink your calories: _____

7. You take small bites and chew, chew, chew: _____

8. You learn what foods are difficult for you and stay away from those choices: _____

9. You always have a plan, each and every day: _____

10. You journal: _____

11. You make yourself a priority. You take care of your health, eat right, exercise, and take your vitamins: _____

Now Be Honest with Yourself about Your Eating Habits

Depending on which diet programs worked for you in the past, you should evaluate which ones you liked and which ones you disliked. How can you incorporate what you have learned in the past to help you on your banded living journey?

_____

_____

_____

_____

_____

_____

_____

_____

_____

_____

_____

If you are a volume eater, the lap band can be your friend. A well-adjusted band can really help with volume—*if* you follow the rules of the band.

If you are a grazer, you need to retool yourself. It will be especially important for you to go back to eating well-planned, high-quality meals each day so that your band can help you with hunger and satiety. If you insist on grazing and cannot break that habit, you should discuss this at your surgical consult.

If you are a die-hard sweets eater, there is debate among the weight loss surgery community about which procedure is best for you. Make sure you discuss this with your surgeon.

If you are a nighttime eater, what is your plan to deal with your habit? Some tips that we've learned include substituting food with a warm, calorie-free beverage, making your bedroom a food-free zone, cleaning your pantry of favorite late-night snacks, and banning eating during nighttime TV.

If you are a binge-eater, you should consider talking with a professional to identify why you binge-eat. The lap band will help restrict the amount of food you can eat at one sitting. It will also slow you down. Again, this is another important topic to discuss with your surgeon. Don't be embarrassed. Your surgeon has heard it all before and wants to help you.

What did you learn from journaling? How will what you learned help you succeed with your band? Many people find tracking their food intake to be beneficial in keeping them on track. Many also find the process of journaling in general to be therapeutic and an important outlet during this often emotional journey.

Exercise 18: Now That You Understand the Lap Band Tool, Summarize What You've Learned (Refer to Exercise 17).

What rules may be difficult for you?

What habits will be most difficult to break?

What other questions do you have for your prospective lap band surgeon about how you will need to use your lap band tool to be successful?

_____

_____

_____

_____

_____

_____

_____

_____

_____

NOTES

NOTES

_____

_____

_____

_____

_____

_____

_____

_____

_____

_____

_____

_____

_____

_____

_____

_____

_____

_____

_____

_____

_____

_____

_____

_____

_____

_____

_____

_____

_____

_____

NOTES

_____

_____

_____

_____

_____

_____

_____

_____

_____

_____

_____

_____

_____

_____

_____

_____

_____

_____

_____

_____

_____

_____

_____

_____

_____

_____

_____

_____

_____

_____

_____

_____

_____

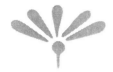

Patty's Story

My relationship with obesity and dieting has existed for as long as I can remember. I could write manuscripts on the topic. I could also travel around the world twice for what I have spent looking for the right diet and solution to the crippling disease of obesity.

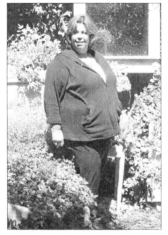

Patty before lap band surgery

What I found to be true for me is that diets don't work. Like a scale, I'd be on one, and off one, only to continue watching my weight go up and up and up! My self-worth was in direct correlation to how much I lost. And if I gained weight, self-loathing would beat me up beyond belief. This got exhausting and humiliating, to say the least.

I was an educated professional challenged with obesity ... why? After years of therapy, diets, nutritionists, fat farms, spas, diet doctors, pills, soul searching, Overeaters Anonymous, losing, gaining, I could not get control.

At fifty-seven years old, it didn't matter anymore. My life was now at severe risk. My health was caving in. I could actually see death on the horizon as the scale tipped three hundred pounds. I thought I knew better than all the doctors out there. I thought I could go on my merry way and weigh three hundred pounds with no effects to my health. The joke was on me.

I had been toying with the idea of bariatric intervention for the five years prior to surgery. I would search the Internet in

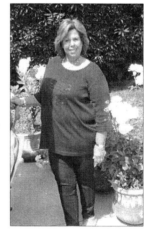

Patty transforming with lap band surgery

the middle of the night, researching and exploring information on surgery. I talked to people all over the States, gathering information from their experiences. I would go to bariatric doctors for consultations. I would go to seminars on the subject. Then panic would set in and I would go back to dieting. I was like a rat in a maze looking for the cheese but with no luck. I continued to spiral downward. Finally, I decided to see a bariatric surgeon who came highly recommended. This was the beginning of my healing. My husband called and set up an appointment to attend a free seminar. As we drove quite a distance to this meeting, my heart was in my throat. I felt so many emotions. There were people starving on the planet, and I was considering surgery to put a device in me to stop the eating. How crazy was that? How crazy was it to be killing myself at three hundred pounds.

Attending this seminar was eye opening. After hearing the surgeon speak, I knew I was home. I made an office appointment to meet with him personally and to have face-to-face explanations and answers to all my questions. His staff, support groups, and patients became my lifeline as I grappled with the decision to move forward. It took me eight more months and continued weight gain before I had lap band surgery.

My life today is so greatly improved since being banded. I feel healthier, with more energy, easier movement, and less medication. My heartburn has disappeared and my blood pressure is close to normal. I sleep well at night. I am now exercising four to five times a week and miss it if I skip a day. Who would have thought this would happen? I have lost sixty-five pounds without gaining it back. This is new and different for me.

The band is my guard dog. It is a tool that reminds me to stay present and conscious when eating. I use mindfulness techniques that support eating less and help me stay connected. My cravings and hunger have been silenced. I check within myself to see if my hunger is my mind speaking or if it is real physical hunger. When I pay attention, there is a difference and an answer. Being honest with myself and my feelings helps. I eat to satisfy the hunger, and if I overdo it, I pay for it. Surrendering to the fact that the band works is the best solution.

I am a work in progress. I still grapple with the obesity demons and work hard to silence the negative chatter. The band is not a panacea.

I still have to do the work to earn results. As my doctor once said to me, gaining the weight back is "like a dry sponge to water" if you don't work a program.

I am grateful for every moment to be alive. I feel a new sense of freedom. I am lucky to have a loving husband of thirty-five years and two wonderful sons. I am surrounded by family and friends. In my heart I feel all of this would have been taken from me without the support of lap band surgery.

Step 5: Attend a Seminar

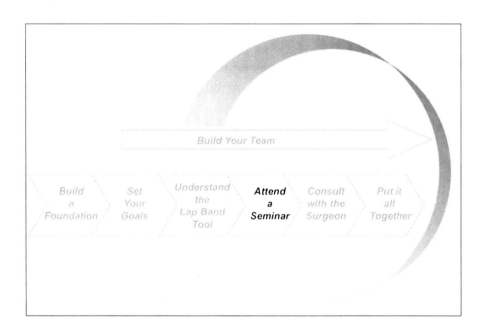

Objective

The objective of this step is to guide you to:

- Decide which seminar you are going to attend
- Prepare to get the most out of the seminar
- Understand your out-of-pocket cost versus what insurance will cover
- Get to know the surgical practice
- Have your questions answered
- Determine if this practice is a good fit for you

Introduction

We have found that many people start exploring weight loss surgery by attending a seminar. That's fine if that's where you started. We encourage you to go through all of the exercises, starting from the beginning of this book, to make sure you haven't missed anything that may be important to your decision or your success.

In exercise 4, you narrowed down your list of bariatric surgeons. Now you are ready to attend a free informational seminar.

The decision to attend a seminar happens in different ways. Sandi was frightened into it by having a blood pressure crisis while in her primary care physician's office. Gloria had tried and failed at her last diet and had been researching weight loss surgery for a while. Your primary care physician, a friend, a coworker, a relative, a newspaper ad, a radio or TV commercial, or, yes, even a billboard may have brought you to this moment.

Whatever your reason or motivator, you have chosen to attend a seminar to learn more about lap band surgery and how it can help you achieve better health and quality of life. Now let's use your time wisely by completing the exercises below.

Deciding Which Seminar You are Going to Attend

Exercise 19: Which Seminar to Attend

Which seminar are you going to attend?

_____

_____

_____

Why?

_____

_____

_____

Practice name	_____
Date	_____
Time	_____
Seminar location	_____
Practice name	_____
Date	_____
Time	_____
Seminar location	_____

Prior to attending the seminar, please review the section entitled Understand the Lap Band Tool.

Do I Really Want to Go through with This?

I remember walking into the room in the dungeon of the hospital where I was immediately surrounded by fat people. I was flooded with the feeling that I really didn't want to be there, but I followed through with it since my husband, Chuck, was willing to come with me and learn about this new procedure. I knew I didn't want anybody cutting or stapling me, but the lap band sounded interesting, if only it would work.

In came two nice looking men in suits. I wondered which one was the doctor because they were equally inept at using the projector. I crossed my arms over my body and sat listening skeptically, trying to find fault with every word that came out of the doctor's mouth. But guess what? I couldn't. He was charming, attentive, honest, and, most of all, really caring. I looked at Chuck and asked him if I should make an appointment. He gave me the freedom to do whatever I wanted and told me he would support me whatever my decision was. How did I get so lucky?

I made an appointment, took home a lot of paperwork to fill out, and began the real work of deciding if I wanted to go through with it.

—Sandi

The Good Student Looking for the Right Answer

On a hot day in Southern California, I attended a free informational seminar. It was a long drive, and I wasn't that familiar with the downtown area. I finally found the building the seminar was held in. It was sweltering in the noon sun. I used to love hot days. Soaked with sweat, I wondered how different the walk from the parking lot would feel if I weren't carrying along all my extra weight.

The seminar was in a large auditorium. The doctor presenting was not the one I had an appointment with. I felt alone and afraid. There were probably seventy-five to a hundred people there. I checked out everyone in the room, comparing who was fatter than me, who was smaller than me. Lots of people brought someone with them. I wished Tom, my husband, was there.

I was the good student, you know the one who sits in the front row and asks lots of questions. I listened intently to every word. At that time, I was leaning toward the lap band, but I still wasn't sure. The audience was armed with lots of questions. The doctor presenting was pretty sterile, and I didn't feel a connection with him.

After the seminar, I had a chance to ask my questions one-on-one. I wanted to know which procedure the surgeon would recommend for someone like me. What I heard in response was basically that neither surgery was perfect but the bypass results were better, and that if the band could deliver the bypass results, it would be a perfect surgery. I didn't understand why he said the bypass results were so much better after just showing us a slide that stated the results were similar. I guessed that his opinion had something to do with seeing his patients more frequently in the first twelve to eighteen months. The other thing that stuck out was that the post-op patients who were at this seminar all had their surgery within the first year. I really wanted to see real live, breathing people who were two, three, or four years out.

—Gloria

Exercise 20:

Based on where you are right now, go back and review the previous sections. Then list at least five questions you would like to have answered, clarified, or to hear the doctor's perspective on.

_____

_____

_____

_____

_____

_____

Investigate and Understand Your Insurance Coverage

Each insurance company is different, and the coverage they offer is different. As a matter of fact, within each company, there are many different plans that offer different coverage. Your best bet for getting a handle on what will be covered by insurance versus what you will be required to pay yourself is to break the cost process into three categories:

- Pre-surgery Testing
- Surgery
- Aftercare

The most important item of note here is that many insurance companies that do cover banding, whether HMOs or PPOs, have requirements that you must follow prior to being approved for weight loss surgery. Make sure you are familiar with them.

The second item of importance is that if you have an HMO, do not begin any pre-surgical testing or visits without their prior approval, even if you know that weight loss surgery is a covered benefit. HMOs all require referrals and have specific referral processes that must be followed to ensure coverage. Please be patient so you don't lose valuable coverage and time.

The insurance coordinator of the practice you choose works with all of the insurance companies and can often answer many of your insurance questions.

Pre-surgery Testing

Each surgical practice will require some testing before a surgical procedure. Every practice has different requirements, and based on your existing medical conditions and age, you may be required to have additional testing beyond the standard testing. For example, many practices require an electrocardiograph (EKG) for their surgical patients. However, if the surgeon determines that he needs more data than the EKG provides, he may order a stress test or refer you to a cardiologist for further evaluation. All of this is done to medically clear you for surgery.

Many of the pre-surgery tests are standard tests, like blood work, chest X-rays, upper GI swallow, and EKG. A visit with a nutritionist, psychologist, and your primary care physician are usually required as well.

Check with your insurance provider to see how all of these will be covered by your plan. These costs are typically not included in the cost of surgery.

Tests, Tests, and More Tests

I was about a month away from my surgery date and was going back to the doctor's office for more pre-op workups. I had lost fourteen pounds since my first visit, and I was still not really cutting out anything, just paying more attention. It really wasn't quite as hard as I thought it would be. At that point I was hoping I was done with tests. I was getting sick of them. I had to sleep with a CPAP machine and oxygen since I was diagnosed with sleep apnea. What a joy that was. I looked like the creature from the black lagoon—how sexy! But who am I kidding—what is sexy about a 424-pound woman in the first place?

—Sandi

Surgery Cost

The cost of lap band surgery itself varies all over the country, so we will not cover the actual dollar amount here, but rather we will discuss how to determine if you have insurance coverage and what percentage of the procedure will be out-of-pocket cost. Do your homework and be sure to include pre-op costs, the costs of the surgery, and aftercare costs. Then you can determine how much your insurance will cover and what will be out of pocket.

You are putting your life in the hands of the surgeon, so you are not shopping for a bargain. You are researching for a skilled, compassionate surgical practice that has experience with this type of surgery and a history of good outcomes.

Contact your insurance provider to find out what their coverage is for lap band surgery. Find out what percentage the company pays and what you are expected to pay. For example, some plans may cover 80 percent and the patient 20 percent.

Aftercare

With lap band surgery, aftercare is a critical component. You will want to know the following:

- The number of visits to your surgeon and the number of fills per year that your insurance will cover. Once again, this varies greatly among insurance companies and specific practices.

- Does your surgeon's office have what is commonly called a program fee? This would cover all of your aftercare for at least one year, if not longer, when not covered by your insurance. If so, how much is the fee? The program fee would be an out-of-pocket expense for you.

Exercise 21:

Call your health insurance customer service line and write down the answers to the following:

Is lap band surgery a covered benefit?

_____

What are the requirements to qualify for covered lap band surgery? (For example, some plans require several months of a medically supervised weight loss program.)

_____
_____
_____
_____
_____

What is my percentage of the cost?

_____

What does the insurance company pay for aftercare visits, and how many per year do they allow?

_____
_____
_____
_____
_____

What do they cover for pre-op testing (blood work, X-rays, EKG, etc.)?

_____
_____
_____
_____
_____

Your surgeon's insurance coordinator should be able to help you determine what out-of-pocket costs will be. In addition, **the manufacturers of the lap bands have resources on their website, along with toll-free numbers to call to help you with your insurance.** They also provide financing options.

Not a Covered Benefit

When I was exploring surgery, I found out my insurance would not cover any of the procedure, so I had to decide if I wanted to do it as a private pay. That led to some other tough questions, like what if something happened during surgery? Would my insurance cover the cost of that?

I couldn't understand why my insurance wouldn't cover this life-altering procedure. The major corporation that provided the insurance to my husband specifically requested an exclusion for bariatric surgery coverage. This corporation made a conscious decision that no surgery for weight loss was to be covered. In addition, they would not cover any surgery for sleep apnea, a condition I had that could be cured by weight loss sustained after a weight loss surgery.

As I pursued this through the ranks of his company's HR department, I was finally told that the procedure does not work, which is why they do not cover it. I asked them if they were willing to pay for all of the co-morbidities that I had and would continue to develop because of my excess weight. They said as long as they were covered benefits, then yes. So, here's the summary: they would not cover weight loss surgery because "it didn't work" but would cover all of my medications, all of my hospitalizations, and all of my doctors visits for any of the conditions I developed due to my weight. It didn't make sense.

Even with all the resistance, I knew in my heart that having the surgery was the right thing for me at that time in my life.

—Sandi

Getting to Know the Surgical Practice (Credentials and Beyond)

Let's say you have chosen to attend a particular seminar because of its location, from a specific referral, or in response to an advertisement of some sort. You can further research the surgeons in the practice with your state or local medical board to find their credentials as well as malpractice suit information. You can also see if the surgical practice has a website, which you should thoroughly review. The surgeon should be a member of ASMBS and be certified by the manufacturer of the band that will be used for your surgery. Additionally, you will want to know if you can feel comfortable as a part of this medical practice, as you will be seeing them frequently.

Assessing the Surgeon

Choosing the right bariatric surgeon may be the most important decision you make. The surgeon who performs your lap band surgery procedure will also be part of your support team for years to come, so it's important for you to feel at ease with him or her. The staff at your surgeon's office will also be an important part of your support team. Your goal is to make sure that you feel well supported by the entire practice right from the start.

Ask Questions

One of your most important roles as a patient is to be your own advocate. This means you need to ask a lot of questions and make sure you feel comfortable putting your life in this doctor's hands. Below are some considerations when choosing a surgeon:

- **Center of Excellence (COE) designation**—COE programs are judged by strict criteria established by the Surgical Review Corporation and the American College of Surgeons. Both of these accrediting bodies do careful office inspections to ensure excellent preoperative and postoperative care specific for bariatric patients.

- **Experience**—Like any other surgery, you want the best surgeon performing your operation, one that specializes in the type of surgery you are having. An experienced surgeon is less likely to have complications on the table. You have a right to ask about the number of procedures a surgeon has performed and the clinical outcome data.

- **Referrals**—Talk to the surgeon's other patients. Patients willing to refer family, friends, and other interested candidates are a good indication of the surgeon's quality.

- **Commitment**—You want your surgeon to be as committed to your weight loss success as you are. He should provide long-term care with follow-up appointments, information, and support resources.

- **Staff**—It's not just about your surgeon. You will be seeing a lot of your surgeon's staff as well, such as the program coordinator, physician's assistant, nurse practitioner, nurse, dietitian, and others. You will work closely with this team before and long after surgery, so it's important for you to meet everyone and talk about how you will work together to help you reach your goals.

Exercise 22:

If you had a magic wand and could list the characteristics of the doctor and staff, what would those characteristics be? (List at least five.)

_____

_____

_____

_____

_____

_____

_____

_____

_____

_____

The Role of Aftercare in the Practice

You want to make sure that aftercare is an important component of the surgical practice you are researching. Aftercare may include:

- Fills and follow-up appointments with the surgeon or staff
- Nutritional counseling
- Support groups
- Trainers or fitness advisors
- Psychologists

Does the practice provide support groups? If so, how frequently do they meet, and is the time workable for you? (Workable means that you can juggle your other responsibilities in order to go once or twice a month.)

Exercise 23:

Call the surgeon's office, get the support group dates and times, and attend one as soon as possible. While you are there, note and write down the following:

Who leads the support group?

_____

Is it specific for lap band patients only?

_____

Are specific topics covered at the meetings or is it just an open meeting setting?

_____

Does the group feel comfortable and safe?

_____

Is there an opportunity to ask questions and share with other patients?

_____

Exercise 24:

In addition to visits with your clinical staff, what other aftercare services does this practice offer, and what have you learned about the practice?

_____

_____

_____

_____

_____

_____

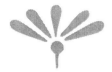

Chris C's Story

My name is Chris, and I was a morbidly obese man who weighed close to 450 pounds before making the choice to have the lap band.

I've struggled with weight my whole life, but around 1999, it got out of control. I got to 300 pounds, then 400 until I reached an estimated 450 pounds. During those years, I always said, I'll start dieting tomorrow, but tomorrow would come and I would break down by lunch time, and start bingeing.

My life had gotten to a point where I could hardly function. I had trouble doing my day to day tasks as a children's pastor. There were times I had to sit at the top of the stairs to catch my breath. I had a hard time breathing when I went to bed...all the fat from my chest would push up and choke me out...I would wake up sometimes gasping for breath. Personal hygiene became an issue. And just about every night, I would stop off at two to three fast food restaurants and load up with a mess of food. It was not uncommon for me to eat a pizza, double cheeseburger, fries, and four to five pieces of fried chicken in just one night. I was out of control.

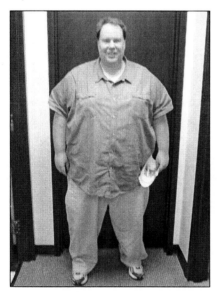

Chris before lap band surgery

One evening about three months before I had the lap band surgery, I hosted a volunteer appreciation dinner at the church where I worked. I was on my feet the entire day getting ready, and of course on my feet the entire evening serving. That night I got home and was in pain that was indescribable. My feet, legs, and back were screaming for relief. I was crying out to God, asking for help as I've done for years, and at that moment I realized that if God gave people wisdom to come up with something like the lap band to help folks like me, then I needed to take advantage of that wisdom. It was at that moment I had peace to have the lap band and decided immediately to get it. That was a Saturday night. The next Monday, I did the research of doctors, fees, preparing for the surgery, recovery time and within three months I got the lap band.

I knew the lap band was not the answer, but just a tool to help me control the amount of food I ate. After getting the lap band, I began to eat healthy and started exercising. In the course of a year and a half, I lost more than 260 pounds, trimming down to a healthy 184 pounds.

If you are struggling with obesity, I would encourage you to do the research to find out if the lap band is for you.

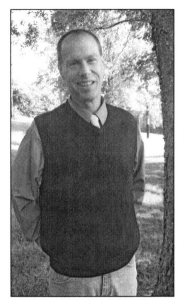

Chris after lap band surgery

Have You Had Your Questions Answered?

Here are the most frequently asked questions at seminars based on our experience:

Q Will my insurance cover this?
A See previous section for answer.

Q How long will I be out of work?
A Typically, doctors recommend the patient take one to two weeks leave from work. If your job is physical in nature, you may require more. Only your surgeon can answer that directly.

Q Will I be hungry all the time?
A For most patients, the combination of having a properly adjusted band combined with smart food choices solves the constant hunger problem. The band helps with portion sizes, the patient helps with choices.

Q What are the risks of surgery?
A While individual risks will vary based on individual medical history, lap band surgery includes the same risks that come with all major surgeries. There are also added risks in any operation for patients who are seriously overweight. For more about surgical risks, speak directly with your doctor and visit the band manufacturers' websites.

Q How much weight loss can I expect?
A Typical results are losing 50 percent of excess weight. Remember, you control the ability to improve these results. You can choose untypical results and achieve 90 to 100 percent loss of excess weight, just like Sandi and Gloria.

Q Will you work with my other doctors who are supervising specific medical conditions?
A This answer should, of course, be yes.

Q Which surgery is best for me?
A This is a personal decision, with the answer reached by a joint decision of doctor and patient and will probably not be made in the seminar setting.

Q Do you have financing available?
A Many practices refer you to Care Credit or other organizations that specifically finance medical procedures. Also refer to the manufacturers' websites.

Q How long will I be in the hospital?

A Lap band surgery is often done as an outpatient procedure. However, some insurance companies may actually require an overnight stay. In addition, a specific preexisting medical condition may influence your doctor into having you stay in the hospital.

Exercise 25:

Make a list of questions you would like answered at the seminar, leaving space to write the answers in later. (Specific questions related to your personal medical history may be better answered in a one-on-one setting.)

_____

_____

_____

_____

_____

_____

_____

_____

_____

_____

Exercise 26:

Is there anyone you want to attend the seminar with you?
Who?

_____

_____

_____

_____

_____

Why do you want them there? (Remember, you are building your team.)

_____

_____

_____

_____

_____

Be sure to bring this book with you to the seminar so all of your questions can be answered.

Determine if this practice is a good fit for you

Exercise 27:

Now that you have attended a seminar and reviewed all of the information, answer the following:

Do you believe weight loss surgery is a good solution for you?

_____

Do you believe you can achieve your goals with lap band surgery?

_____

If you brought someone with you, what questions and feedback do they have?

_____
_____
_____
_____
_____

How are they influencing your decisions?

_____
_____
_____
_____
_____

Do you want to see the surgeon whose seminar you just attended? Is this surgeon a good fit to be on your team? (Refer back to the section entitled Build Your Team.)

_____
_____
_____
_____
_____

How many surgeons are at the practice? Will the surgeon presenting the seminar be the one performing your surgery? If not, when do you get to meet the surgeon?

_____

_____

_____

_____

_____

Does this practice offer aftercare that meets your needs?

_____

_____

_____

_____

Did you meet anyone else at the seminar whom you would like on your team?

_____

If yes, record his or her name and contact information.

_____

_____

_____

_____

_____

Are you comfortable with the surgical practice? Is it time to schedule a consult?

If you are not comfortable with this specific practice, consider attending a seminar sponsored by another surgical team. If you choose this option, please review the entire Attend Seminar section before going and insert additional notes for the questions you have remaining to be answered.

NOTES

NOTES

NOTES

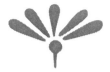

Meg's Story

Istruggled all my life with my weight. My father was killed when I was only five years old. This left my family devastated. I turned to food; my mom and brother turned to alcohol and drugs.

When I was only seven, I began sneaking food. By the time I was old enough to drive, I was eating fast food all the time. Over the years I tried everything. I would find willpower, read weight loss books, try different diets, and lose some weight only to regain and then some.

I found myself at 350 pounds. Every visit to my doctor would wind up being a discussion of my weight with me blaming my obesity on everything and everybody. I would blame my mom for being a drunk or my dad for abandoning me, but in truth, it was me. I was eating myself to death. I was the one making *my food choices*. Food is an addiction for me. I would have massive cravings for McDonalds every day; some days I would eat both breakfast and dinner there. I had terrible cholesterol and triglyceride levels and was diagnosed as pre-diabetic. I could barely walk around my apartment because of severe knee pain.

Meg before lap band surgery

On January 4th, 2010 my life changed. I went to a seminar on lap band surgery. I took my mom with me. The surgeon did not sugar coat anything. She said if you're going to do this you need to be committed 100 percent and do the work. I had a bit of soul searching to do, but deep down I knew this was the solution for me. It was permanent, and doctor guided. This surgeon was going to help save my life. I was so excited!

My primary care doctor had been recommending the surgery to me for two years. I was stubborn and thought I could do it on my own. Who was I trying to fool—the doctor or myself? I was approved quickly as my weight, co-morbidities, and diet history were well documented. As excited as I was, I was also terrified. Could I do this? Would it work? Would I stay committed? Did I want to really change, or was I too afraid to change? I had my lap band surgery on March 24, 2010—my re-birthday.

This is a big change for me and so far, I'm doing really well, one day at a time. I have to be willing to follow my surgeon's guidelines—she calls them her "rules" and she means that!

Five months into my journey, I have lost a total of eighty-four pounds, a bit more than half way to goal. I see my surgeon monthly and call if I have any questions or issues. I have had no problems with the band thus far. I am so happy that I had the surgery and would do it all over again in a heartbeat. I've already had so many victories: I can fit in my car with my stomach far away from the steering wheel now; I can walk for a few miles with minimal pain in my knees; I am more outgoing and upbeat; I am making plans for my future because I know I have one; I am making new friends—we support each other; my food is very healthy and I have nothing in my house that would sabotage my way of eating.

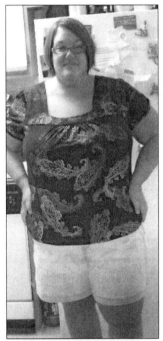

Meg transforming with lap band surgery

Because of my surgeon, her staff, support groups, and support online, I am saving my life daily! I make a choice each day to do the right things. This is finally *my life*! I am doing things now, taking pictures, and building memories!

This is by far not the end of my story. I know I will reach my goals because I make the decisions in my life now. I am learning all about self love and unconditional love by putting myself and my needs first, more often than I ever have before. I am learning who I *really* am and I'm starting to like me.

Step 6: Consult with the Surgeon

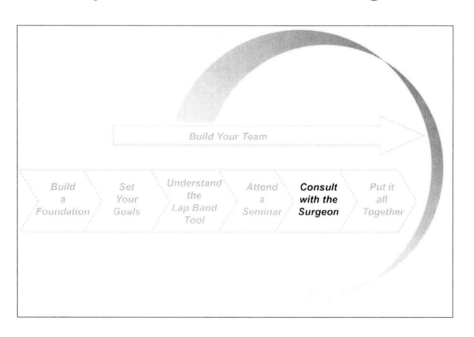

Build Your Team

Build a Foundation → Set Your Goals → Understand the Lap Band Tool → Attend a Seminar → **Consult with the Surgeon** → Put it all Together

Objectives

The objectives of this step are to:

- Prepare for your consult
- Assess the surgical practice
- Plan your next steps

Introduction

You have now built your foundation of information, set your goals, begun to understand the lap band tool, and attended a seminar. You've scheduled your surgical consult. That's a big milestone. You can get the most from your consult by coming prepared. Since you have attended a seminar, you already know a lot about the practice, the surgeon, and his or her staff. Now you are ready to meet for that one-on-one time.

Prepare for Your Consult

You probably have paperwork to complete before your consult. It looks like a lot of work, but much of the information you need has already been collected in this book. Don't wait until the day of the visit to complete the paperwork. Answer questions with as much information as possible in order to help the doctor, the insurance company, and, in the end, yourself. If you've made it this far, you are seriously considering lap band surgery.

Decide if you are going to bring a member of your team to this office visit with you. If yes, who will it be?

_____

_____

_____

_____

_____

Deciding to Take Control

I remember my first appointment with my surgeon. It was just like every other medical office. I had to wait almost an hour in the waiting room. Then my six-foot-two husband and I were squished into a six-by-six examination room with a doctor who was six-foot-five. My 424 pounds filled up the rest of the free space in the small room. I went through my ideal weight (137 pounds), realistic goal weight (200 pounds), and the accomplishments I hoped to achieve with the doctor.

I had been fat since I was a kid. My pictures at four years old are of this chubby child. And those chubby pictures continued until I was sixteen and went on a diet with a diet doctor, taking pills, shots, and probably no more than 800 calories a day. I eventually became a size eight and weighed 135 pounds. Boy, did I look good for the five minutes I held that weight (for one summer, actually). I explained to the doctor how I had been up and down in weight ever since that summer. I was ready for help.

After the preoperative screening, the doctor suggested that gastric bypass would be a good surgery for me. His opinion was that because of my size, I would have definite results with bypass, whereas he could not predict if I would follow the rules of the lap band. However, the procedure did involve some major changes in the stomach and intestines. Nope, I didn't want to be cut and stapled—I wanted a lap band. It was just a device that went around my stomach, could be filled with fluid to make it tighter, and could be easily removed if I hated it. The surgery took less time and posed fewer potential risks.

We went through the things I wanted to change about my life by having weight loss surgery, like the ability to interact with my family and the freedom of movement. I realized at this visit that I had been existing in a world that was diminishing in size and quality due to my self-inflicted incapacity. It was time to finally gain control!

—Sandi

There are many steps to take after the initial consult until surgery. The doctor or his or her medical staff will review them with you at this initial visit. They may include any or all of the following:

- Medical clearance
- Blood work
- Imaging (GI)
- A sleep study
- EKG or other cardiac clearance
- PCP clearance
- Psychological screening and clearance
- Nutritional consult
- Insurance approval
- Pre-op visit and testing
- Pre-op classes

Exercise 28:

Review your book and plan to bring it with you to this visit.

Review your goals in terms of health, weight loss, and quality of life. List any changes:

_____
_____
_____
_____
_____

What are your biggest health concerns about weight loss surgery?

_____
_____
_____
_____
_____

What lifestyle changes will you need to make?

_____
_____
_____
_____
_____
_____
_____
_____
_____
_____

What are you concerned will be your biggest challenges?

_____
_____
_____
_____
_____
_____

Is there anything in your history that may become an issue (e.g., eating disorders, compulsive behaviors, history of abuse)? If so, you must discuss these with the doctor. Remember, he (or she) has heard it all before.

_____
_____
_____
_____
_____
_____
_____
_____
_____
_____

Is this a bad time in your life to sign up for lap band surgery (e.g., you're planning on getting pregnant this year; you're getting married in three months; you're moving to another part of the country)? Life will always have its ups and downs. However, there may be certain events or significant issues that would drastically reduce your odds of achieving your goals.

_____
_____
_____
_____
_____

Be sure to review all of these questions at your first consult.

Finding the Right Match

I spent months researching surgeons and completing preoperative testing. Dr. Billy wasn't the first surgeon I consulted with. I wanted to find the right fit—someone who I felt completely comfortable with. I remember my first appointment with Dr. Billy. His waiting room was packed. I liked the energy there. Waiting for my name to be called, I remember feeling pretty sure I wanted the lap band. I waited with a bit of anticipation, and then my name was called. It was finally my turn. First things first, they took my weight. I weighed in at 225 pounds. I hated scales. I'd hated them for as long as I could remember.

When I met Dr. Billy, he didn't look anything like the picture I had seen on his website. It must have been an old picture, I remember thinking. He was about six-foot-five and close to my age. He was someone I could be friends with. I really liked him. He was honest, direct, and smart. I could picture myself coming to that office every month.

After listening, I mean really listening to my story, and doing a thorough exam, he told me that he thought I was a good candidate for weight loss surgery. He wanted to make sure I'd done my homework about the surgery and about him. I think he was worried that I might be jumping into this too quickly. I asked Dr. Billy which surgery he recommended for me and why. He said I would do really well with the lap band, and would only do a bypass on me if I felt very strongly about it and could explain my reasons. I liked that he was willing to offer an opinion. I asked how quickly he could do surgery if I wanted to proceed. He said that if I was paying with cash and my medical records were in order, it could be within weeks.

I called my husband, Tom. He encouraged me to get Dr. Billy's first available date. At that time, I had no idea how important my choice of surgeon would be. That was the beginning of a very important relationship. Over time, I realized that Dr. B was really my head coach in my battle to win back my life.

Sitting on the side of the road parked outside the Target shopping center with cars whizzing by, I scheduled my surgery for August 16, my husband's birthday. My husband's birthday ended up being the first day of the rest of my life.

—Gloria

Exercise 29: Unanswered Questions

Review your book and list any questions that you still have and would like answered at your consult. Leave space to write in your answers. Don't worry about how many or how few you have. Everyone in the practice should welcome questions, as this shows your participation in the process.

_____
_____
_____
_____
_____
_____
_____
_____
_____
_____

_____
_____
_____
_____
_____
_____
_____

Assess the Surgical Practice

Now you have made it through your first surgical consult and have met the doctor and his or her team.

Exercise 30:

Soon after you leave the office, think about the following:

Were all of your questions answered?

_____

If not, what questions do you still have?

_____
_____
_____
_____
_____
_____
_____
_____
_____

If you brought a member of your team, what is his or her feedback?

_____
_____
_____
_____
_____

Did you feel comfortable and safe with this doctor and his or her team?

_____
_____
_____
_____

Do you want this practice as part of your team? Is this a place you can come back to month after month?

_____
_____
_____
_____
_____

Was the office warm and inviting?

_____
_____
_____
_____

Do you have any other concerns? (Include your gut reaction.)

_____
_____
_____
_____
_____
_____
_____
_____

Decide What Your Next Step Is Going to Be

We hope your first consult went well and that you found the surgeon you are comfortable with to start you on your journey. Congratulations. You are ready to put it all together.

If this practice does not feel like the right fit for you, you may want to consider interviewing another surgical practice or attending a seminar offered by that practice if that is an option for you.

NOTES

NOTES

NOTES

_____

_____

_____

_____

_____

_____

_____

_____

_____

_____

_____

_____

_____

_____

_____

_____

_____

_____

_____

_____

_____

_____

_____

_____

_____

_____

_____

_____

_____

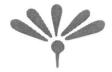

Janet's Story

Where do you start when writing about something that is so life changing that it encompasses literally every aspect of your life? In the beginning growing up as the middle child in a family of five girls you can imagine the emphasis put on clothes, looks, weight, etc. I was not fat; I had to keep up with my gorgeous sisters. In grade school I enjoyed playing sports, and was always of an acceptable weight.

So when did my serious weight problem begin? It began as an adult. My husband and I were married, had a baby and bought our first house all within one year's time. I was working full time and adjusting to marriage, a new baby, and new responsibilities all at once. It was an extremely exciting time and busy time. With a demanding career, I most definitely did not have the time or energy to spend at the gym working off that baby weight. Baby number two came just seventeen months later. My greatest joy is being a mom, and I love everything that goes with it. I was not willing to spend what little free time I had at the gym when I needed to be with my babies. My weight only increased after the second baby and continued to increase. An already out-of-control weight issue only got worse. Suddenly, I found myself obese. I was too busy living my life and taking care of everything and everyone else. Obese was an unbelievable word to me.

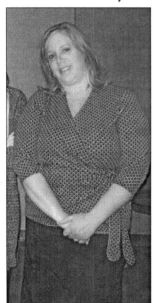

Janet before lap band surgery

I tried every diet in the book. Each failed attempt seemed to only make the problem worse. I would lose and then gain back more than I lost. That discouraged me and lead to depression and lack of energy, neither helping me on the road to recovery. Working in the medical field, I hear about new upcoming therapies and treatments all the time. I asked my doctor about the lap band. She was very discouraging, telling me that I didn't need to do anything so extreme. I could just diet and exercise as she had done after having kids…yeah right. That only made me feel like a failure. So I continued with my struggle, tried more diets, and the problem continued to grow.

At the time, my favorite companions were other moms with small children, working full time and living very full, busy lives. I became friends with some very amazing women. One in particular was Gloria the author of this book. She trusted me enough to tell me that she was considering lap band surgery. I watched Gloria's journey—from making the decision to having the surgery, to the follow-up work and ultimate success. Shortly after, I began a new position at the very company that makes the LAP-BAND® System device. I was very interested in having lap band surgery, but secretly wanted to see how Gloria did before I made the leap. One day Gloria sent me a picture; I couldn't believe the transformation. If I had any doubts at all, they were gone once I saw that picture and how successful she was. Not long after that, my company made it impossible for me **not to** have the surgery; they offered it free for all employees. I was the first to sign up and I haven't looked back since.

The first thing I learned from Gloria is that the lap band is just a tool. You still have to put in the work. I had to remind myself of that a lot, as my weight loss was not fast. I lost my 80 lbs. over a period of two and a half years. Yes, I had to work, but that was not discouraging in the least. I saw results! Slowly but surely, I was becoming fit and healthy again! I did not hide the fact that I had the surgery. Everyone saw my progress. It's not easy to accept compliments and answer questions, but the look of amazement on other people's faces always brought me back to reality. I was actually changing for the better! I eventually began to believe what other people were saying—I actually looked good, more importantly, I felt good! I reached a plateau and was really struggling until I realized I had to step up my workout routine. So I started boot camp. Who would have ever thought that I would partake in boot camp? I did, loved it, and lost even more weight. I'm healthier now than I have been in a long time. I owe it all to the lap

Janet after lap band surgery

band, my friend Gloria who inspired me to take that first step, and doing the work and putting in the effort so that this amazing "tool" will continue to work for me!

Step 7: Put It All Together

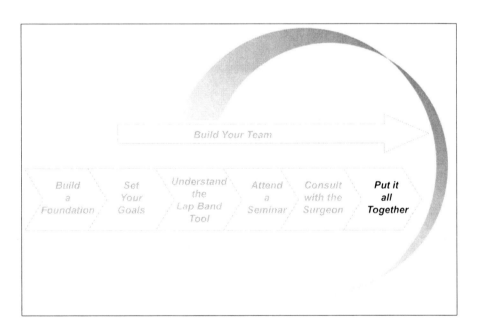

Objective

The objective of this final section is to bring together all of your work to answer the question:

- Is lap band surgery for me?

Introduction

You now have a basic understanding of weight loss surgeries, you have set and redefined your personal goals, you have some understanding of what the lap band tool is all about, you have attended a seminar, you have an idea of what your insurance will cover, and you have visited the surgeon's office for your initial consult. Now, how do you put this all together to help answer that big question?

Foundation

Do you meet NIH guidelines for weight loss surgery?

_____

If not, what was the outcome of your discussion with the surgical practice?

_____
_____
_____
_____
_____

Do you meet your insurance guidelines for weight loss surgery?

_____

What costs are you going to have to pay out of pocket? (Be sure to include costs of aftercare.)

_____
_____
_____
_____
_____

Team

Do you have the right team to support you on your journey?

» Loved ones

_____

» Primary care physician

_____

» Bariatric surgeon

_____

» Other patients

_____

» Friends and colleagues

_____

What concerns do you have about your team? What is your plan for dealing with those concerns?

_____
_____
_____
_____
_____

Are there new members of your team that you want to start actively recruiting at this stage of your journey?

_____
_____
_____
_____
_____

Goals

After reviewing the book, reassess your goals by reviewing step 3 and step 6.

Now summarize your health, weight loss, and quality of life goals by listing them below again. Be sure to think through all the information you've collected, especially your discussions with your doctor and his or her team.

Health

_____
_____
_____
_____
_____

Weight Loss

_____
_____
_____
_____
_____

Current Weight: _____

50% Excess Weight Loss: _____

Your Goal Weight: _____

Quality of Life

_____
_____
_____
_____
_____
_____
_____
_____
_____

Understand the Lap Band Tool

Do you understand how the lap band tool works?

_____

Do you understand what restriction is?

_____

Do you understand what you will need to do to use the lap band as a tool? (Refer back to exercise 17.)

_____
_____
_____
_____

Do you understand what changes you will need to make to accomplish your goals?

_____
_____
_____
_____

Which changes will be most challenging for you, and what is your plan for handling those challenges?

_____
_____
_____
_____
_____
_____
_____

Do you have a plan to accomplish your goals?

_____
_____
_____
_____
_____

Attend a Seminar and Consult with a Surgeon

Have all your questions been answered? If not, what questions still remain, and how are you going to get those questions answered?

_____

_____

_____

_____

_____

_____

_____

_____

_____

Have you thoroughly discussed the risks and complications with your doctor based on your unique medical history?

_____

_____

_____

_____

Are you prepared to visit this practice frequently, month after month? This is like a marriage, for better (weight loss) or worse (weight gain)?

_____

Does the aftercare program meet your needs?

_____

_____

_____

_____

_____

Have you been completely honest with your doctor? (Understanding that we have all faced the shame and embarrassment surrounding the issues of obesity.)

_____

_____

_____

_____

_____

_____

_____

_____

Is this a good time in your life to sign up for lap band surgery?

_____

_____

_____

_____

Are you emotionally equipped for lap band surgery? Is there anything in your history that may become an issue (e.g., eating disorders, compulsive behaviors, history of abuse)? If so, will you be seeking professional help? Have you discussed these with your medical team?

_____

_____

_____

_____

What else are you worried about?

_____

_____

_____

_____

You've done your homework. Is lap band surgery for you?

If yes, why?

_____

_____

_____

_____

_____

If no, why?

_____

_____

_____

_____

_____

Regardless of your decision we need your feedback to help others. Please also answer the following:

How did this book help you with your decision?

_____

_____

_____

_____

_____

What was most helpful to you?

_____

_____

_____

_____

_____

What suggestions do you have for us to make this book more helpful?

_____

_____

_____

We'd be grateful if you would please take a moment to log onto www.bandedliving.com and share your feedback with us. On the top of our homepage, click on forums and locate the "Is Lap Band Surgery for Me" forum and post your feedback there. Thank you! Good luck on your journey.

—Sandi and Gloria

Useful Websites

The following websites may be useful during your weight loss journey, along with brief descriptions of what the individual site has to offer:

www.asmbs.org

This is the website of the American Society of Metabolic and Bariatric Surgeons. The vision of the society is to improve public health and well-being by lessening the burden of the disease of obesity and related diseases throughout the world. The site contains information about surgeries, benefits and risks, and current information about new studies, and has a specific section for patients.

www.bandedliving.com

This is the official Banded Living community website for lap band patients by lap band patients, regardless of where they are in their journey.

www.calorieking.com

This website provides free detailed nutritional information for thousands of foods, including menu items at popular restaurants.

www.fitday.com

This website provides free detailed nutritional information for thousands of foods.

www.gloriasbandedliving.com

This blog contains the story of Gloria Samuels's journey from 232 pounds in 2006 to 145 pounds in 2007 through lap band surgery. Gloria continues to maintain her healthy weight and shares her experiences, triumphs, and setbacks including how she uses her lap band as a tool in real life with her blog followers.

www.lapband.com

This is the website of the manufacturer of the LAP-BAND® System.

http://www.ncbi.nlm.nih.gov/pubmed/

This site is commonly referred to as PubMed, which comprises more than 19 million citations from Medline, life science journals, and online books. Citations may include links to full-text content from PubMed central and publisher websites.

www.obesityactioncoalition.org

This organization brings together and acts as the voice for individuals who are facing the often lifelong battle with obesity.

www.obesity.org

The Obesity Society is a leading scientific society dedicated to the study of obesity.

www.realize.com

This is the website of the manufacturer of the Realize band.

www.sandisbandedliving.com

This blog contains the story of Sandi Henderson's journey from 424 pounds in 2004 to 174 pounds in 2006 through lap band surgery. Sandi continues to maintain her healthy weight and shares the tips, successes, and setbacks of daily life with a lap band with her audience.

www.win-niddk.nih.gov

This is the government's weight-control information network, which provides the general public, health professionals, the media, and Congress with up-to-date, science-based information on weight control, obesity, physical activity, and related nutritional issues.

Bibliography

Publications

US Department of Health and Human Services, National Institutes of Health, National Institute of Diabetes and Kidney disorders, Weight Control Information Network (WIN)

- 2009. Bariatric Surgery For Severe Obesity, NIH Publication
- No. 08-4006

Brethauer, Stacy. Chand, Bipan. Schauer, Philip.

- 2006. Risks and Benefits of Bariatric Surgery: Current Evidence. Cleveland Clinic Journal of Medicine 73: 1–15

Brethauer, Stacy. Goncalves, Carolina. Cummings, David. Rubino, Francisco. Kaplan, Lee. Kashyap, Sangeeta. Schauer, Philip.

- 2009. Bariatric Surgery as a Treatment for Type 2 Diabetes Mellitus in Obese Patients, Obesity Management 5(3): 112–118

Levi, Jeffrey. Vinter, Serena. St. Laurent, Rebecca. Segal, Laura.

- 2010. F as in Fat: How Obesity Threatens America's Future 2010, Trust For America's Health, Robert Wood Johnson Foundation

Websites

- American Society for Bariatric and Metabolic Surgery, <www.asmbs.org>, (July 2010)

- CalorieKing—Diet and weight loss. Calorie Counter and more <www.calorieking.com>, (July 2010)

- Obesity Action Coalition, <www.obesityaction.org>, (July 2010)

- The Obesity Society, <www.obesity.org>, (July 2010)

- The Preferred Weight Loss Surgery | LAP-BAND®, <www.lapband.com>, (July 2010)

- REALIZE® Solution, <www.REALIZE.com>, (July 2010)

- The Weight-control Information Network, <www.win.niddk.nih.gov>, (July 2010)

About the Authors

Gloria Samuels is a highly successful lap band patient and mentor to bariatric surgery patients. Having experienced the life-changing benefits of bariatric surgery—a ninety-pound weight loss maintained since 2007—she is passionate about giving back and helping others learn to conquer obesity. Gloria is using her prior experiences in the corporate world to build the Banded Living community to educate, advocate, and provide hope for all who struggle with significant weight issues.

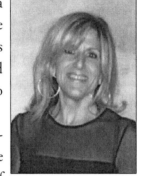

Before launching Banded Living, Gloria enjoyed a successful twenty-six-year career in corporate America as an executive and officer in some of the world's most respected corporations. Gloria served on the board of directors of a public company and has been the recipient of several industry awards, including *Computerworld's* Premier 100 IT Leaders.

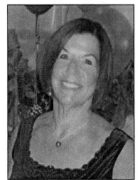

Sandi Henderson is extraordinary in the world of lap bands having lost 250 pounds since her surgery in May 2004. She started with a BMI of 68.5 and has maintained her weight loss since 2006. She has been interviewed both on local TV and national newspaper regarding her success with lap band surgery. Sandi mentors both new and prospective surgery patients. She is passionate about helping people understand there is a solution to obesity, and works tirelessly to advocate and set an example for others.

Prior to the launch of Banded Living, Sandi had a successful twentyone-year career as the owner and chief operating officer of a computer business. As the COO of a small, woman-owned company, she has done business with the federal government and other public sector entities, as well as in the private industry, including many of the Fortune 500. She has been featured in magazines such as *Diversity Business* for her success in a highly competitive market.

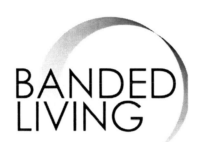

Index

C

calorie
  calorie 65, 82, 83, 84, 86, 101
  calories 12, 19, 62, 63, 82, 84, 85, 100, 138
calorieking.com 83, 161
candidate
  candidate for lap band surgery 11
  candidate for weight loss surgery 13
cardiologist 116
Center of Excellence
  Center of Excellence ix, 38, 120
  COE 38, 120
challenges 5, 139, 156
chemotherapy 16
colleagues 3, 154
colon 22
comorbidities
  comorbidities 119
  resolution of comorbidities 15, 55
complications
  complications 2, 19, 21, 22, 49, 77, 120, 157
condiments 84
consult
  consult xii, 128, 137, 138, 140, 141, 144, 153
  consultation 3, 29
  surgical consult 101, 137, 142
Coronary 12
counseling 38
coverage
  coverage 116, 117, 119
  insurance coverage 14, 37, 117
CPAP
  CPAP 117
  sleep apnea 6, 117, 119
cravings 108, 132

D

deaths 13
dehydration 49
diabetes

diabetes 14
  Type 2 diabetes 12
diet
  diet 16, 17, 62, 72, 77, 78, 86, 100, 101, 107, 113, 133, 138, 148
  diets 3, 53, 77, 107, 132, 149
dietitian 120
digestion 22, 79
duodenal switch 18, 22

E

EKG
  EKG 116, 118, 138
  electrocardiograph 116
Ethicon Endo Surgery
  Ethicon Endo Surgery 25
  Johnson & Johnson 25
EWL
  EWL 61, 78
  excess weight loss 61, 78, 81
exam
  exam 35, 87, 141
exercise 17, 38, 62, 63, 72, 77, 82, 85, 100, 113, 149, 156
expenses
  cost 11, 113, 116, 117, 118, 119
  expenses 14
exploring lap band surgery 4
eyes wide open vii, 53

F

failure v, 78, 149
family 1, 3, 34, 37, 48, 54, 56, 65, 66, 109, 120, 132, 138, 148
FDA ix
fill
  adjustment 85
  fill 80, 81, 85, 114
fitday.com 161
followup

36, 37, 39, 40, 48, 49, 54, 57, 61, 62, 73, 80, 84, 86, 101, 107, 113, 115, 116, 117, 119, 120, 125, 126, 127, 128, 133, 138, 141, 149, 153, 165

weight loss surgery i, 14, 37, 77, 80, 138, 139

T

testing
  testing 116, 118, 138, 140
thirst 81
tighten
  adjust viii
  fill 80, 81, 85, 114
transformation 62, 149
tummy tuck
  plastic surgery 49
  tummy tuck 49

U

unbanded 80

Urinary incontinence 12

V

Venous 12
vitamins 22, 82

W

walking 6, 65, 114
website
  website x, 18, 118, 119, 141, 161, 162
  websites 11, 24, 37, 83, 125, 161, 162
weight loss
  weight loss i, viii, xi, 1, 5, 14, 19, 20, 21, 22, 23, 37, 53, 57, 62, 63, 67, 77, 79, 80, 81, 86, 119, 120, 125, 132, 138, 139, 149, 154, 157, 165
  weight loss surgery i, 14, 37, 77, 80, 138, 139